MARRIED WITH CANCER

One Couple's Journey

Eileen and Jimmy Newell

Edited by
Janet Angelo of INDIEGO PUBLISHING

Cover Design by
JudithSDesign&Creativity
www.judithsdesign.com

Book Formatting by
Amit Dey

Paperback ISBN – 9781946824288
Hardback ISBN – 9781946824295
Ebook ISBN – 9781946824301
LCCN – 2018952424

Published in the United States of America
INDIEGO PUBLISHING
www.indiegopublishing.com

Publisher's Cataloging-In-Publication Data:

Names: Newell, Eileen. | Newell, Jimmy, 1950-.
Title: Married With cancer : one couple's journey /
Eileen and Jimmy Newell.
Description: [Florida] : IndieGo Publishing, [2018]
Identifiers: ISBN 9781946824288 (paperback) |
ISBN 9781946824295 (hardback) | ISBN 9781946824301 (ebook)
Subjects: LCSH: Newell, Eileen--Health. | Newell, Jimmy,
1950---Health. | Breast--Cancer--Patients--Family relationships. |
Lymphocytic leukemia--Patients--Family relationships. |
Cancer--Patients--Care. |
Married people. | Caregivers.
Classification: LCC RC262 .N49 2018 (print) |
LCC RC262 (ebook) | DDC 362.196994092/2--dc23

MARRIED WITH CANCER

One Couple's Journey

THIS BOOK *is* DEDICATED TO

Sean, Jeannine, and Bryan

We have been blessed in so many ways, but none so special as having three wonderful children. You are the reason we are able to have such joy in our lives.

We love you very much.

Mom and Dad

CHAPTERS *of our* JOURNEY

How This Book Was Born

My wife Eileen and I have been married for over forty years. We have three children. We raised our family on the east end of Long Island in the area known as the Hamptons. For much of that time, I commuted on the Long Island Rail Road more than five hours each day. For her part, Eileen worked even longer days as a nurse at various area hospitals.

Like most families, we've had our good times and bad, but we have faced life's challenges together. In the year 2000, I was diagnosed with chronic lymphocytic leukemia (CLL). To this day, I am not sure I have ever accepted this diagnosis, though I certainly have had every reason not to be in denial.

Part of my inability to grasp the significance of my diagnosis was that I really didn't feel sick, so I played it down and even joked about it. I was concerned about the reaction Eileen and my children would have as well as the rest of my family, and I thought that if they saw me acting as I always had, they would be reassured that it wasn't that big a deal.

To be honest, however, I don't know what I was thinking that first day when I got off the phone with my primary care doctor when he gave me the news. I immediately called Eileen and dropped the bombshell on her, and, try as I might to play down its serious nature, she knew better, even if I did not.

Ten years later, when I came home from work on a beautiful summer evening in July of 2010, I got to experience what it felt like for Eileen to receive such shocking news. As soon as I walked in the front door, she made me sit down because she needed to tell me something. This was odd, and I immediately sensed something was wrong. I had no idea just how wrong.

She sensed my dread and got right to the point. She told me that she had breast cancer, and it was bad.

What I learned at that moment was something Eileen had understood during my diagnosis and treatment: It is never easy being the patient, but being the caregiver has its own challenges because it makes you feel helpless to watch your loved one suffer and not be able to wave a magic wand to make it all go away.

In the pages that follow, Eileen and I will share how we dealt with our own cancer and each other's. Our journey hasn't always been easy, but sometimes we've had fun, and most times we've had boundless love that has brought us closer than when we were newlyweds. There have been tears and laughter, and a few life lessons that we never thought we'd have to learn.

It seems appropriate that we started writing this on National Cancer Survivor's Day, June 2, 2013. We celebrated that day by attending a meeting of cancer survivors at Southampton Hospital in Southampton, New York.

The day started with a discussion of what comprises a cancer survivor. The broadest definition includes not just the cancer patient but also the patient's entire team — family, friends, and health care providers. For Eileen and me, the size of our combined team is staggering. It continues to grow.

The next thing I learned was that I was embarrassed listening to the stories of the panelists who offered their experiences with cancer as a patient and as a survivor. I had it so easy compared to many of the people who spoke, as well as those in the audience who nodded their heads in agreement.

When I think about what my wife endured during her treatment, and what she continues to endure, I feel kind of silly and ashamed thinking about the times I felt sorry for myself.

I also learned a new mantra: "Victor, not victim."

I vowed to live up to the concept of being a victor, and to leave the victim behind. I should have learned that lesson from Eileen, but I have been known sometimes not to listen.

The other thing I learned was that Eileen and I have a story to tell. We started talking about it before we attended the meeting, but Eileen got a head start at 3:00 a.m. that morning. An idea for the title of a book we planned to write came to her, but we decided that His Story Her Story: A Couple's Guide to Survival seemed a bit cumbersome, so *Married with Cancer* was chosen for our title.

The concept of this book grew the more we talked about it. Each of us would write about our own cancer, but we would also write about each other's so that we were both writing from the vantage points of patient and caregiver, and ultimately, survivor.

I was the patient first, and I never knew how hard it was being a caregiver until it was my turn. Eileen's writing from her viewpoint as a patient gets right to the heart of the matter, whereas I have a tendency to worry more about how I write rather than what I write. I hope that my writing is an equal match to the poignancy and emotion in hers.

Though we may differ in style and, at times, subject matter, I think we have accomplished our purpose for writing this book — to illustrate the importance of family, friends, and healthcare providers who make you feel it is their life's mission to make your day. We also hope to reveal the intimate moments of joy and pain, struggles and small victories of being a married couple with cancer.

I never would have imagined going into an oncologist's office and being happy to see the people there — one of the many hidden blessings of this path that Eileen and I are walking together day by day.

We hope that our story will encourage others waging their own battle of survival.

Love At First Sight

We met on the Friday night of Labor Day weekend in 1971. Eileen was seventeen and I was twenty-one. I didn't care about the age gap because I fell in love the moment I laid eyes on her. The same was true for Eileen, and not a week went by after that first meeting that we were talking of building a life together.

Some people might hear this story and think that we were just a couple of cute kids who knew nothing about making a life-long commitment, and we were caught up in the moment of starting a new relationship. Maybe that was true, but you couldn't convince us otherwise, and time would prove us right.

I was finishing my degree at St. John's University while Eileen was finishing high school at St. Helena's, but we were already making plans for the future. I wanted to be a high school teacher, and was planning to go to graduate school. Eileen wanted to be a nurse and had her heart set on St. Vincent's School of Nursing.

If there were one thing to describe our relationship as Christmas 1971 approached, it would be laughter. I loved to make Eileen laugh. She lit up like a Christmas tree when she smiled, and when she laughed — well, you couldn't help but laugh right along with her.

As you might imagine, a seventeen-year-old girl dating a twenty-one-year-old man was a bit scandalous in the eyes of an Irish Catholic family. But even a concerned family could see how deeply Eileen was in love with me, and after only a little while they could see that I would take good care of her.

We spent long afternoons talking and walking and planning. Often we went to Macy's in Parkchester in the Bronx where I would soon learn that beige was Eileen's favorite color that year.

While we dreamed in the jewelry section and picked out a pearl ring that would be my Christmas present to her, we quickly saw the wisdom of a more practical, less romantic gift, and so a nice watch was pointed out and later purchased.

On a subsequent visit to the store, I shopped alone and purchased the watch as well as a beige sweater, glove, and hat set. It would be another year before that pearl ring graced Eileen's hand.

And so, Eileen and I studied and worked and saved and planned. Though it was a long five years for us, we eventually kept the promise we both silently made to ourselves on a subway ride a mere two days after meeting in 1971.

On September 19, 1976, at Blessed Sacrament Church, in a Mass and ceremony witnessed by our family and friends and presided over by Father Pat Carrol, Eileen and I exchanged our vows.

Of course, all journeys have their bumps along the way.

When we were planning our wedding, Eileen gave me specific assignments while she took charge of her own duties.

I looked for an apartment.

I looked for the limousines.

I did very little else.

Eileen, on the other hand, had her hands full with all the details of the wedding and reception, not to mention the bridesmaids' dresses and flowers and on and on and on.

She also wrote our vows.

You see, in 1976, it wasn't enough to leave the vows to the priest. The couple had to bear witness to their love and express their serious devotion to each other by writing their prosaic and heartfelt testimony of their love for one another.

I never asked to see our vows. Eileen gave them to me at the altar.

At the appropriate time, when Father Pat asked us to express our intentions, Eileen began by reading a beautiful statement of her love for me, and her desire to share a life with me for the rest of her life.

It caused me to mist up ever so slightly, but it was enough.

Then as my vows were to be read, I picked the cards out of the vest pocket of my rented tux and began reading.

"Grant us, O Lord, these wishes..."

Well, that is what I should have read. What I really proclaimed to all present was:

"Grant us, O Lord, *three* wishes..."

Father Pat was forced to cover his microphone so the congregation wouldn't hear his roaring laughter.

Despite this seeming setback, Eileen and I were married and began our life together.

We moved into our apartment in Flushing after a relaxing and romantic honeymoon in Bermuda. Flushing was a convenient location for Eileen to commute to St. Vincent's Hospital in Greenwich Village and for me to finish my graduate work at St. John's.

Eileen graduated from St. Vincent's School of Nursing in 1975 and immediately started working in one of their orthopedic units. Not surprisingly, her first exposure to St. Vincent's was in the same unit, but as a patient when she was seventeen years old just a few weeks before we met. Now, she would be a nurse, and perhaps she might encourage a patient to consider nursing as a vocation, much as she had been inspired.

Even though it was a short subway ride into midtown Manhattan, often times I would drive her to work and, more importantly, drive her home when she worked evenings.

Eleven o'clock at night was no time for a young woman to ride the New York City subways alone.

I learned early on not to get to the hospital right when her shift ended. If she was on the three to eleven shift, I knew better than to be there at eleven. Maybe I would leave Flushing at eleven, but even then, I would arrive at the hospital and wait a while because Eileen never left when her shift was over. For Eileen, the shift was over when her work was done. Couple that with a nursing shortage, and sometimes she didn't come out to the car until around midnight.

There was no union at the hospital. No overtime was ever paid. Eileen was grateful to make a difference in her patients' lives, and she gave them as good a hospital experience as possible. That's just the way it was for her. Forty-three years later, she is still that way.

Meanwhile, I traveled to mid-town where I worked for the National Football League.

Having worked for the City of New York Department of Human Resources only to be laid off during the city's fiscal crisis when President Ford "told" the city to drop dead (actually, he merely denied the city's request for a financial bail-out), I was forced to return to my mail clerk roots. The following year I achieved my dream of being a teacher.

Although teaching in a Catholic school paid about the same as a mail clerk in the NFL, the pride of being a teacher was its own reward.

St. Vito School in Mamaroneck, New York, was an ideal place for me to teach. Possessing the perfect mixture of a dedicated lay faculty guided by a group of nuns and priests who bucked the stereotype of severe and strict authoritarians that neither laughed nor tolerated fun, St. Vito's would become my Garden of Eden.

Oh yeah, St. Vito's had students, too, and the students were what I loved most about teaching.

I was lost during the summer when school was not in session. The first day of school was like New Year's Day, something to celebrate and not bemoan. The looks on my students' faces and the sound of their groans every time I made a bad joke, and I made many, delighted me to no end.

Although I was only there four years, it was enough to make more life-long friends than I could count. More importantly,

I acquired the skills that any father worth his salt would need to raise a family.

Life was good, but it wasn't always joyful.

Pain and suffering are part of life, and just when things seemed to be going along smoothly, Eileen's brother Patrick succumbed to Hodgkin's disease. Then, a little more than two years later, my mother, whom we affectionately called Lizzie McHugh (her first name and maiden name), was taken from us.

However, each loss was soon followed by a gift. The first came not long after Patrick left us.

Having moved to New Rochelle in the fall of 1979, we both worked in the area and set out on a course that would eventually bring us to East Quogue on Long Island.

In the fall of 1980, Eileen and I were on our way to an Elton John concert in Central Park. On the subway heading into the city, Eileen expressed a feeling that she might be pregnant. Well, that feeling was enough to derail any plans to attend a concert with a hundred thousand people pushing and shoving against my wife.

The stress was too much for me to contemplate, so we scratched our day in Central Park and substituted it with a trip to Greenwich Village.

Once there, at a drugstore on the corner of Sixth Avenue and Eighth Street, Eileen purchased a pregnancy test. We may have had lunch that day, but I can't remember. I was beside myself with anxiety. I just wanted to get home and find out once and for all if we were pregnant.

We were, of course, and Sean was born in my last month of teaching at St. Vito's School. The dream to teach would eventually have to be discarded, superseded by the practical reality of supporting a growing family. Although we were able to pay our bills, we had dreams of owning a house and moving out to the Hamptons. Making eight thousand dollars a year as a Catholic schoolteacher just wouldn't cut it.

I was a dad now, and life's decisions were made in a new world of responsibility. And so I cast myself out of St. Vito's School, my Garden of Eden.

Eileen returned to work soon after Sean was born, and we both took turns being the parent on duty since I worked during the day, and Eileen worked the evening shift at New Rochelle Hospital.

I would soon be persuaded to once again work with and for my great friend Mike O'Connor at Columbia University. Not too long after I started at Columbia, my mother passed away. But then our second gift was provided.

It seemed to be a matter of weeks after my mother passed that Eileen told me she was going to have a baby.

This was exciting news and came just as we were planning to buy the house in East Quogue. We closed on the house in October, and Jeannine was born just a few months into the new year.

Now, the only problem with life had to do with the Long Island Rail Road.

My friends and family are excused from reading this section, as I am sure they are sick and tired of my non-ending lament of my terrible commute. It really was terrible, but I did my best to make the most of it by reading and listening to my Walkman and maybe having a cold one on the ride home.

For Eileen, the isolation of the east end of Long Island necessitated weekend trips to the Bronx to see her mother and sister and brothers. My father and brother also lived in the Bronx, so going into the city to visit family was a great way to spend a weekend.

But life brought other opportunities and challenges.

I wanted to go back to school to enhance my career, and hopefully, to find a position on Long Island.

Having been encouraged by my great friend PJ Howley, who had just graduated from law school, I decided to give that a try. The result was a change in our family's living arrangement that would last four years.

Pop, my father, was still living in the Bronx when I decided to attend St. John's School of Law in Jamaica, Queens.

When we first told Pop that we were moving all the way out to the farthest end of Long Island, he was not happy. It was only four months since my mother had died, and our moving so far away must have seemed like we were abandoning him.

During the conversation, he asked how I was going to make a living out there. When I told him that I would take the train into the city to work, he immediately responded, "Don't think you'll be staying here with me." I could tell from this response that he really was struggling with deep sadness over my mom's death, because it was not like him to say this, and as it turned out, I did exactly that.

To this day, my memories of going to law school and living in the Bronx with Pop are very special to me. You see, by then, the

Prodigal Son was welcomed back with open arms and a fatted calf in the form of late-night dinners and a hearty breakfast every morning.

I have no doubt that living with my father added years to his life because my coming home at night gave him something to look forward to and live for, and we bonded during that special time when it was just the two of us. One night I kissed him when he had a big corned beef sandwich waiting for me when I got home. That made him smile and say, "Momma would be happy."

So, from Monday through Thursday, I went to work in the morning at Columbia University in Washington Heights, and in the evening, I went to St. John's in Queens and then back to Pop's in the Bronx. For four years this routine kept me hopping while Eileen held down the East Quogue fort.

A few weeks after I finished my second year, Eileen presented me with a small gift box on Father's Day.

Not really too sure what to make of such a small box, I opened it to find a plastic toy baby inside. It took a while for it to sink in, but I finally realized that another baby was on the way.

So, three days after my last final for the fall semester of my third year of law school, Bryan was born, and our family was now complete.

This was how our young family started, much like many families, perhaps like yours.

There were celebrations and tearful goodbyes.

There were successes and failures.

There was financial struggle and wealth beyond measure.

Whatever we enjoyed or endured, we did it together.

So it was that cancer entered our lives.

The Yankees, A Physical, And Leukemia: Some Vacation!

Ever since my brother Michael suddenly and mysteriously got ill and died, Eileen was pushing me to take better care of myself. Now she was after me to get a physical to set her mind at ease and reassure her that all was well.

In the year 2000, I turned fifty. I did not want a party or even a gift. So, in celebration of having made it to the half-century mark, I gave myself a gift. I finally made an appointment for a physical. My appointment was August 10.

It's not that the actual physical was so memorable, but it just so happened that my son and I went to see a Yankees game two nights before, and that was extremely memorable. The Oakland A's were in town, and it was Barry Zito pitching for the A's facing Roger Clemens. As it turned out, neither pitcher figured into the outcome of the game, but both pitched pretty well.

The A's had the upper hand as the Yankees entered the bottom of the ninth. Trailing 3-2, the Yankees would be sending Bernie Williams, David Justice, and probably Luis Polonia, who had pinch run for the DH, Glen Allen Hill. It wouldn't matter, as Polonia would never get up to bat.

The A's closer, Jason Isringhausen, the former Met, came in the game to shut down the Yankees. He never broke a sweat, nor did he even come close to shutting down the Yankees. Isringhausen's first pitch to Bernie Williams caused an eruption in the half-filled stadium when the ball was promptly deposited in the right field seats. The save was blown, and the game was tied.

That fact hardly made an impression on the Oakland pitcher as his second pitch, this time to David Justice, nearly brought down The House That Ruth Built. I have heard crowds roar, but never like that night as David Justice hit a walk-off homer to give the Yankees the win. The teams would meet again in the playoffs, but this was as exciting a game as any I had ever seen.

I tell this story because it helps to re-create my state of mind for that week in August 2000, a week that would change my life and the lives of all who love me.

I was off that week, and even though submitting to a physical exam was not as exhilarating as a thrilling walk-off win at Yankee Stadium, I felt good about doing something that needed to be done, and I would still be able to spend a nice vacation day at the beach.

Blood work was drawn, a chest X-ray taken, and the dreaded prostate exam confronted and endured.

So far, so good.

My doctor told me that the blood test results would come back in a few days, so I felt relieved that I had at least that amount of time to enjoy what would probably be my last steak and cheeseburger, never thinking that my cholesterol numbers would be the least of my concerns.

But I was cruising. It was summer, and the living was easy.

My vacation ended abruptly, as they often do, when I set off for work on Monday, August 14, but the long train ride was pleasant because the only thing on my mind was the Yankees. I was still basking in a happy glow from that game.

Work was proceeding better than it had the previous year because our computer system finally was working the way it was supposed to — almost. At least I wasn't constantly peppered with questions about when the student loans would be coming in. You would think that working at a college would be less stressful than, say, trading on Wall Street, but you'd be wrong — very wrong.

I wasn't even thinking about the results of my physical that Monday. We were in the midst of our busy season at my school, which is to say, it was a normal day of students and parents calling and trying to navigate the heavy seas of financial aid.

Things were not nearly as bad as the previous summer when we were implementing a new computer system that resisted implementation. That year — when everyone was scrambling to reprogram computers to accept 20 on the front of years instead of 19, the dreaded Y2K, as it was called — had me frazzled beyond anything I had experienced since practicing law. The president of the university called me every morning at 8:00 a.m. to ask how we were doing and when the loan money was coming in.

But on this particular Monday, things were running rather smoothly, and my angst level was nonexistent.

Then, the phone rang. My secretary said my doctor was on the line, which was very unusual.

Life Is A Puzzle

Minutes before the doctor called, I had looked at the calendar and noted that it was nearly three years to the day since my brother Mike first got sick in August 1997.

I was thinking about that day because it began just like this one, but then my mind drifted back to the following year in August 1998.

That month ended one of the most distressing years for my family and me. It was, in fact, a distressing year for anyone who knew my brother Mike. On August 26, 1997, we lost my brother, and it seemed I relived that loss every day of the year that followed.

But, on the anniversary of his death, in August 1998, something happened to make me smile and shake my head in wonder and amazement, and things began to get better.

In order to set the mood for what will follow, I must go back to the day of his funeral Mass. For some reason, I felt that I had to give the eulogy. Although some of my friends and family may not believe it, I was never comfortable getting up and talking in front of a crowd. The prospect of giving my brother's eulogy was not something I had wanted to do, but I felt compelled to say goodbye and to represent everyone who loved him.

One of the things that struck during the days and nights of his wake was the huge turnout of people who came to pay their respect. They were waiting outside on Castle Hill Avenue for over an hour to get into the funeral parlor. My friend Paul asked if Mike had been a Pope. There were so many people there that it was hard to grieve. The crowd overwhelmed us and made us realize that Mike wasn't just special to his family; he was beloved to all who came in contact with him. It reminded me of George Bailey in the movie *It's A Wonderful Life*. In fact, I used that in my eulogy.

I also quoted a line from *The Wizard of Oz*. I said, "In *The Wizard of Oz*, the wizard tells the tin man that a heart is judged not by how much you love but by how much you are loved by others. Mike had a magnificent heart."

Many of you know that I love Lionel trains and have a considerable collection. I blame Mike for this. He had me loving Lionel trains just like he had me loving Mickey Mantle and the Yankees, and Joe Namath and the New York Jets. Sometimes Mike made mistakes, but we always loved our Jets.

One time a few years before he died, I told Mike that I saw a beautiful Santa Fe locomotive. Unbeknownst to me, the next day he went to the train store. He called me when he got home and said that he saw the engine and put a $50 deposit on it for me. He said, "You just have to get it." From time to time when I am searching for trains on eBay, I still hear that voice, and it takes me right back to 1994 and my brother's thoughtful gesture.

I started my day on August 26, 1998, like I did most days. I called Margaret, Mike's wife, and we talked and cried like we did every other day, and we both said that sometimes it felt like twenty years or just last week since Mike left us. I then went about my work and had a typical day talking to students and pushing paper. Then before I knew it lunchtime had arrived. I always do the *New York Times* crossword puzzle at lunchtime, and this day was no exception.

I started the puzzle and was going along pretty well for a Wednesday when I came to a clue that had me smiling and shaking my head. "Name of Famous Train," six letters. It was amazing because the answer was Lionel!

I immediately called Margaret and told her of this terrific coincidence. She said, "He's watching you, Jimmy."

I continued the puzzle, and then a clue or two later came upon "Eulogizes." The answer was Lauds. I gave his eulogy! Can you believe this? Now it was getting freaky. I called Margaret again and she was amazed.

This crossword puzzle had a clue for an answer that spanned the entire puzzle going across. I hate those because it's usually something I am not familiar with like Greek mythology. I couldn't avoid it any longer, so I read the clue. "Frequently aired movie." I was hyperventilating. I was sure it was *It's a Wonderful Life*. It wasn't, and I was kind of upset. It would have made a nice trifecta and a great story. But then I had another thought.

Sure enough, *The Wizard of Oz* was the correct answer. Mike was there, and he was messing with my head. I called Margaret and we were both speechless, but we knew what we felt was true. Mike was with us.

That puzzle was sacred to me, and I stopped doing it upon entering *The Wizard of Oz*. I never went back to it. I put it in my bag, and there it remained until the summer of 2002.

We were getting rid of our van, and as I was cleaning out the back seat, I came across my bag. I took it out and reviewed its contents, and saw the puzzle. I began telling a neighbor the story of the puzzle just as I have outlined it here for you. I added that I never went back to the puzzle, and as I said this, I noticed another clue: "Brooklyn Sch." The answer for this, as those of you who do the puzzle should already know because it is a repeater like Bobby Orr, is LIU. One of the campuses of LIU was Southampton College where I had just recently started working.

Believe what you want, but no agnostic, atheist, or whatever kind of nonbeliever exists can convince me that this life is all there is. The puzzle of life and death has, for me, been solved by another puzzle, and while I got neither a job nor my faith through the *New York Times*, I sure got a strong editorial of its support that only the clueless would deny.

It's amazing how a memory can flit through your mind when something in your life takes you back to a time that made an indelible imprint on you. My thoughts had gone through this time-warp loop just before my doctor called, and he was waiting for me to answer the phone.

I don't remember his exact words, but the underlying tone indicated there was something very wrong, and in fact, there was a problem with my blood cell count, but for some reason, that didn't sink in.

I did hear the words "leukemia" and "good kind."

He had to repeat the condition that I had, and I wrote it down as he spoke: Chronic lymphocytic leukemia. He also told me that very often patients with CLL live a long, normal life and die of natural causes or something else.

As soon as I hung up the phone with the doctor, I called Eileen.

I guess I was in shock. You hear the word leukemia, and the words chronic or good cancer really don't register with you. I only knew that leukemia killed people. In fact, Eileen's father died of leukemia when she was a year old. Now I had to tell her that her husband had the same disease.

I used the same tact that my doctor had shown me. I was reassuring. I told her that if you had to get cancer, this was the one to get. I really believed this at the time because I didn't feel sick. I was actually thinking the diagnosis was a mistake because I didn't feel any different than I had in the last ten years.

The phone call to Eileen went something like, "I just got off the phone with my doctor, and I have chronic lymphocytic leukemia" — said in a very casual, offhand manner like it was no big deal. Who was I kidding? I probably even mispronounced it, but she knew.

I told her that it wasn't that bad. She said she would contact the oncologist that my doctor had recommended, and that was that.

Then I hit the internet.

What I didn't know was that Eileen was shocked by this news, scared, and despite my best efforts, not one bit reassured.

I'll let Eileen tell you.

"I ran to the nursing office to compose myself because, as a supervisor, I had to maintain composure. I needed to think, to take it all in. I looked at Jimmy's numbers and reflected on the implications. Then I looked up CLL. As a medical professional, I knew what it meant, but now it was personal. I wanted to make sure that what I remembered about CLL was correct. Then my nurse's training kicked in. Nursing had taught me to be prepared and to have a plan. So, I started to plan.

"But what I learned is that you can get ahead of yourself and add to your sense of insecurity. So, I decided to take it one step at a time: first, the oncologist. I made the appointment. Oncc that was set, who should I call next?

"In a matter of seconds, my role was shifting. Wife. Mother. Nurse. Now, Caregiver was added to my list.

"At this point, the Big Unknown was front and center. I had to face it. I had to make friends with it. It wasn't going away, so I had to embrace this new challenge.

"I felt a little more in control. That was huge, even if it didn't last. I had a moment of control — another lesson learned. Take what you can from every moment if it helps you."

The first time I read what Eileen has just shared was while I was revising this section of the book. I never knew what she just described. I knew she called the doctor and set up my appointment, but I never knew she had all this going on.

I, on the other hand, sat in my office staring blankly at nothing, taking in this new information, not sure what to do next.

Now, everyone will tell you don't go to the internet when you get this type of news because no good can come of it. You'll suddenly have every symptom of every horrible disease out there. I did read that CLL was a chronic form of leukemia and that many people lived a full, normal life, often without going through any treatment whatsoever. However, like my doctor indicated, nothing about CLL can be guaranteed.

People still die.

The word cancer is scary enough. But I have to say that the word leukemia frightened me and made me numb at the same time. I think numb quickly turned into denial. Eileen might agree with this. Instead of getting all freaked out about my diagnosis, I immediately went back online and found "good" things to say about leukemia. I was in damage control mode.

I was also worried about having to tell people. I didn't want to scare my family and friends. Looking back, I was probably the one I didn't want to worry. So I found terms like "the good cancer" to affirm my no-big-deal attitude. I read that many people with CLL never get treatment, and that most die of other causes.

What really happens is you realize that being in control is the best position to be in, so you hunt for and arm yourself with information so that you can ask your doctor all the questions running through your mind, and before you know it, you are managing your fears.

That initial conversation with Eileen set in motion a flurry of activities, but it was Eileen, being a nurse, who went into action.

She identified the oncologist/hematologist that I would consult, and I had an appointment to meet with him later in the week.

Life is funny.

Here I am given what most people would consider bad news, and the first thing I think of is being worried about asking for another day off. I had just come back from vacation, and I had to take another day off. How many other days would I need? How crazy am I that I was obsessing over taking a day or two off? Again, maybe that was a way of not thinking about cancer and leukemia.

I am sure if you ask cancer patients, many will tell you that they had an instinctive desire to keep the news of their diagnosis to themselves. I have heard from others that they didn't want their boss or company to know about their illness because they didn't want to jeopardize their job.

That's not how it was with me. I immediately told my boss. I put her on notice that I had cancer and that I would need to take time off for tests and appointments. She said the right thing. "Do whatever you have to do."

That's what I did. I did what I had to do, but the whole time I was thinking, *We'll see how well that works out.*

I also told my staff and colleagues, and I was lucky because I had a great staff and they were extremely loyal to me. They still are even though I no longer work there. My boss was reassuring. My staff had my back, so I had no worries concerning work.

Now I had to tell my kids.

Michael's death was such an emotional loss for me, and also for my children. They never saw me cry as much or as often as the day he died and the entire year following his death — every day, and that is not an exaggeration. I would get to the train station early, and while awaiting my train, I would just break down even if it was only a minute. Then, when I called Margaret, I would cry some more.

I thought of all this as soon as I hung up the phone from telling Eileen about my diagnosis. How was she going to survive my death? How would my children? Of course, I never voiced these concerns and went about my life as normally as I could. I joked and laughed, and all the while I never was quite sure if I was fooling anybody, let alone myself.

One of the positive things about working so far from home was that I had time to cool down. By the time I got home, the trials and tribulations of the day were long forgotten, and I rarely allowed them to interfere with my real life. Work was not my real life. It was a means to an end, an intrusion on my real life, something that had to be tolerated during workday hours before living my real life at home.

To a certain extent, I was able to do this with my diagnosis. I was able to compartmentalize my life so that chronic lymphocytic cancer was left in the driveway when I got out of the car to come into my home. Well, of course that first night I had to deal with Eileen's reaction to this news, but I never let her see the fear and uncertainty that hid behind my poker face. Surprisingly, I somchow managed to allow my poker face to shield me from her worried looks too. I saw what I wanted to see. I felt what I wanted to feel. I didn't break down or indicate how scared I really was.

I pride myself on being an upbeat kind of guy. I have a great sense of humor, and I am very funny. Well, I am my biggest fan, and I am not sure if others think I'm as funny as I think I am, but I do inspire the odd laugh or two.

I was determined that this would not change because of leukemia. By this point in my diagnosis, I was referring to my disease as CLL, explaining that C stood for chronic, and chronic implied that it wasn't that serious. Denial can be an ally, if only for a short time.

But I couldn't be in denial where my kids were concerned. At some point, I had to tell them, but one of the obstacles I faced in telling my children was the timing of it all.

Sean was nineteen, Jeannine was sixteen, and Bryan was eleven. Sean was due to leave for his second year of college. Jeannine was going to Ireland the very next day. Bryan was of course still living at home with his mom and me.

Telling them that I had cancer was not going to be easy, and each child presented different issues to take into consideration.

Perhaps my biggest concern was that a short three years earlier, they had lost their uncle, my brother Michael, to a mysterious illness when he was only fifty-three. Now, their fifty-year-old father was telling them that he had cancer.

Eileen and I decided that we would not tell Jeannine until she came home from Ireland.

Sean, however, was going back to Fordham University at the end of the week, and I had to tell him before then. You don't want to have that kind of conversation on the phone if you can help it.

We also had to tell Bryan, as he could not be kept out of the loop, even though he was eleven, and he would be upset if we delayed telling him. Besides, he was the only one at home with us until Jeannine came back, and he would figure out that something was going on with me taking days off right after being on vacation.

I decided to tell them separately. I wasn't sure how they would take the news, and I wanted to give them the privacy to react in their own way. Eileen was there when I told each of them, and she was able to put things into context and tell them the truth without scaring them.

You know, kids are amazing. I couldn't tell whether Sean or Bryan were really upset. By all appearances, they were fine and seemed to understand what was going on. Perhaps, because we were forthright and laid out what was going to happen, they were able to process the news with a minimal reaction.

It was years later that I learned otherwise. But, for now, they were fine.

I then had to face the prospect of telling the rest of our family. Eileen's brother Patrick had died of Hodgkin's disease in 1979. Eileen's father died of leukemia when she was a year old. Telling her family that I had leukemia was not going to be easy.

I really had to play up the "good" part of CLL for my siblings.

Side note: I realize that most CLL patients get really annoyed when they hear people refer to CLL as the "good" cancer, but that's how my primary care doctor described it to me, and I used it to soften the blow when telling my family.

Once all the people that mattered had been brought up to speed on my diagnosis, I was ready to face the beast.

But just as I had gotten through the ordeal of speaking to everyone, Jeannine came home from Ireland. This was going to be a tough one. Telling the boys was harder on them than I thought. They seemed to understand that it wasn't "that big a deal," which is how I tried to portray CLL to them, and they seemed to be able to move on. I didn't know that they'd had their own little meltdown.

While Sean and Bryan were able to conceal their true reactions, Jeannine was not. I knew that it was going to be hard on her, but I had a plan.

I was going to be an idiot, and I would keep it up for years.

I made a joke of it all. I guess I figured that if I laughed at CLL, so would she. I found out years later just how stupid I had been and how angry I had made her when I did this. Oh well, no one ever said CLL makes you smart.

One of the things I learned quickly as a CLL survivor is that the internet was both a blessing and a curse. Even before I called Eileen with the news of my diagnosis, I went online to learn what CLL was. I didn't learn anything that my doctor hadn't already told me, and while there was a note of optimism in much that I read, there was also plenty that concerned me.

It seemed that the good news was the ten-year survival rate. Well, I guess that was good news, but I really wasn't thinking about dying in ten years when I got to work that morning. And now, the thought of having ten years remaining was supposed to make me happy?

What I hadn't read that first day was the different experiences that people have with this disease. It's not the same for everybody.

I soon signed up for an email listserv that I read every day without fail. I read accounts by long-term survivors who never had chemotherapy and warned others to stay away from that treatment at all costs. The W&W method, or watch and wait, was preferred over chemicals.

There was a feeling that treatments did nothing to extend lifespans and that the chemicals did more harm than good.

I didn't know what to think.

When I met with my oncologist and had a bone marrow biopsy, I listened to him as we discussed my options. I felt he was someone I could trust. After all, Eileen had known him for a number of years having worked in an area hospital where he practiced.

Additionally, he had a professional demeanor that inspired confidence, and it was very easy to rely on his expertise and defer to his recommendations. Ultimately, we decided to treat my CLL, but I still read my listserv every day, hungry for every straw of hope and bit of information I could grasp.

It soon became apparent that listservs and other sites on the internet offered numerous opportunities to learn. The most important thing I learned, however, is that you can't always trust what you read.

Most of us have realized by now that just because something is written on the internet doesn't mean we should act on it. Back in 2000, it wasn't always that clear. Trust your health care providers over someone who posts a comment or recommendation on the internet. If you can't trust your health care providers, get new health care providers.

The First Thing You Lose Is Your Dignity

On the day of the physical, I was prepared for most of the tests and procedures: chest X-ray, blood test, blood pressure check, urine sample — no problem. But I hadn't prepared for the prostate exam.

When the doctor instructed me to get off the examination table, turn around, and drop my pants, well, I had no idea what was coming.

I soon found out with a little lubricant followed by an invading finger that seemed to stay in just a bit too long.

I guessed at the time that's what happens when you get old. You lose all sense of dignity. Little did I know it was going to get worse.

A bone marrow biopsy was scheduled, and I had the good sense not to ask Eileen what this involved. I was put in an examination room with my oncologist, a nurse practitioner, and Eileen. Once again, I was advised to drop my pants. Actually, I only lowered them a bit, but enough to expose the "hip" which included my ass.

Fortunately, this was the only pain I endured during the procedure because they numbed my hip really well.

I now realized that I had to get over myself and do what had to be done. Pride and embarrassment had to be checked at the door.

Nevertheless, when I saw the size of the biopsy needle, I soon cared less about any loss of dignity and focused on the spear about to pierce my butt.

Another indignity struck when I was almost through my fifth course of treatment back in January of 2001. For the most part, I had handled the chemo pretty well. I rarely was nauseous, and the few times when I was, I only had mild discomfort, nothing that required a mad dash to the bathroom.

But on this occasion, I would have sold my soul to have a need to make a mad dash to the bathroom. I don't usually talk about potty stuff, but this story is illustrative of just one of the concerns when you are under treatment.

One of the more uncomfortable side effects that I suffered during my first chemotherapy treatment was constipation.

I was very uncomfortable, and nothing got things moving. Coffee. Bran muffin. No relief. Finally, I tried laxatives and then stool softeners. (I even hate typing the words stool softeners!)

This went on for several days, and I was in pain. So, I did what anyone would do who is faced with such a challenge. I asked my wife to get me an enema. She thought I was kidding — actually, she hoped I was kidding.

The next day I stayed home from work and went to the drugstore early in the morning. Yes, I had decided to make this an all-day event in case anything went awry.

I went to the appropriate section in the drugstore and immediately wished I could get this dreaded device on eBay. Well,

I could've, but that would've meant waiting for it to be shipped, and I couldn't go another day with this misery. So I persevered and brought the item to the counter to pay for the enema.

Of course, that was not the end of it (if I can use that expression).

When I got to the counter, the clerk took my item and called back to someone, "Hey, Charlie, are we still having the buy one get one free on the enemas?"

I wanted to run out the door screaming, but I really needed the enema.

I was instructed to go back and get a second enema. I didn't want to argue and continue this dreadful experience any longer than I had to, and I could see that the six people in line behind me felt the same way. Besides, for all I knew, it might take two of these bad boys to get things moving. Better safe than sorry.

Finally, I got home, and one thing led to another, and I was feeling better.

However, in my haste to get out of the bathroom now that the deed was done, I left the box and the instructional brochure, complete with diagram, on the counter.

As luck would have it, my daughter Jeannine used the bathroom after me, and moments later, she ran screaming out of the bathroom and into her bedroom, slamming the door to make sure I got the point.

I guess the very idea of one's father using an enema is traumatic to a teen girl. It probably took days to get that image out of her mind!

I learned a valuable lesson, though. Hydration is very important, and I had not been drinking enough water. It's very important to understand the expected side effects you might experience due to any drug that you take. Find out what you can and make sure you let your health care team know if you experience anything out of the ordinary, even if it is not listed as a side effect for your particular drug.

My mother was the wisest person I ever had the good fortune to know. She quoted Shakespeare when she sent my brother and me off to bed when we were kids. "To bed to bed. There's a knocking at the gate."

I was in my junior year of high school when I read that line in Macbeth.

She also had her own sayings, which her mother probably shared with her.

Lizzie was always telling me, "Don't let little things bother you." This was largely what "Don't sweat the small stuff" was all about.

Then there was, "Too much of anything is good for nothing," which is a more elegant way of saying, "Moderation in all things."

The most relevant to my experiences coping with CLL treatments is, "What's good for one thing is bad for another."

This has been the case for me relative to the treatments I have endured over the years. Fleudara greatly reduced my white blood count and really attacked the CLL in my lymph nodes and spleen, and shrunk them in no time. However, it weakened my body's ability to ward off infection. Mepron, an antiviral, was ordered to help fight opportunistic infections. Later on, Rituxin and Fleudara reduced my white blood count to nearly zero.

Currently, I am taking Ibrutinib, which has been such an effective drug in terms of fighting my CLL, but it has had its own share of side effects. Body aches and muscle spasms have affected me. However, the most unsettling is what it has done to my hair.

I have always had very straight hair. My entire life, there wasn't a bend in any hair on my head, and I had no difficulty parting my hair and keeping it relatively flat to my head. Now, I have a curl to my hair.

It's not just any curl. It's a Superman curl. You know, the curl that our superhero has on his forehead? Well, mine is in the middle of my head, on top of my head.

I can't brush it out. I can't plaster it down with any gel or spray.

Then, when my hair gets long enough to require a haircut, it starts curling up everywhere on my head. The sides, curly. The back, curly. And, like their brother on top of my head, they have no interest in laying flat.

The haircutters that I frequent all know about me and my curls. On one occasion, I had three women working on my hair at the same time. Each observed and recommended a course of action. There were notes about me in their computer system.

I know I shouldn't complain because there are so many, like Eileen, who lost their hair due to chemotherapy.

These few minor indignities that I have faced and endured are blessings in disguise. The therapy worked, and I am here to share my embarrassments and laugh at my good fortune.

Jimmy's Treatment

When you begin any treatment, it would be most unusual if you were not apprehensive at the start. I was petrified. But of course, I didn't let anyone know that.

Once we decided that I would have to go through chemo, I soon began the first of six courses of Fludara and Cytoxan.

I would do an infusion every day for five days, and twenty days later, the second course, and so on.

My weekly chemo routine consisted of driving sixty miles to work, arriving around 8:00 a.m., and working until around 1:00 p.m., then driving nearly seventy miles to my oncologist's office to "see the nurses," the euphemism for going in for chemo.

A CBC (complete blood count, as Eileen would instruct me) was done, and then the infusion would begin. I was only in the chair for about an hour.

I usually got home around 5:00 p.m. and, quite honestly, I vegged out downstairs in my man cave until dinner.

For me, the good news was that the chemo worked.

My lymph nodes shrank, and my white blood cell counts dropped to a more normal range. Each CBC indicated that the chemo was working, and I began to rebound so that by the end of the sixth session in February 2001, I was put on a monthly schedule for a doctor's visit and CBC.

The only medication that I continued taking was Mepron to help me fight infections.

By the end of the winter, I really felt normal. I took my kids to Yankee games in late May, and we went on a two-week vacation to Disney as soon as the school year ended for Jeannine and Bryan.

I continued to do well for six years, but in March 2007, during a normal three-month check-up, my oncologist asked how I was feeling. I said my throat was a little sore.

Dr. Avvento always remarked at the size of my tonsils. I don't think he ever saw tonsils as large as mine. On this day, he took one look down my throat and ran out of the room. He immediately came back with Prednisone and a prescription pad. He was very concerned that my tonsils were so enlarged that they were obstructing my airway.

He immediately ordered a tonsil biopsy, and so my second round of treatment was put into play.

Eileen came with me to the tonsil biopsy, and thank God she did. I was sitting upright in a chair similar to a dentist's chair when the doctor approached me. Eileen was on my left and the doctor on my right. Well, they appeared to have changed places for some reason, and I thought it odd that they did.

Then I heard the doctor say, "There he goes."

Well, it seems that they never really changed places, and what I had thought was a momentary nod of my head was a bit longer. I had passed out.

As Dr. Avvento had already surmised, the biopsy showed that my tonsils were filled with CLL, so this time I would be treated with RF, Rituximab, and Fludara.

Rituximab is a monoclonal antibody that doesn't harm healthy cells as much as chemo does. Again, six courses were ordered, and it did the job.

This time I made sure to hydrate before and after each session, and I drank lots of water, every day.

As with my previous treatment, I continued my usual workweek schedule of going in early so that I could leave early to go to chemo. I did this for four of the five days. The first day of Rituximab was always a long day and a slow infusion, so I was not able to work those days. This created tension for me at work.

One of the things that happened to me when I got cancer is that I was almost immediately scared of losing my job. I know how employers can be. If you're sick and forced to take time off, you are not a valued employee. I am ashamed to admit that I allowed a couple of people to let me feel that way.

Here I was going through a life threatening experience, and I had a guy wonder how I was making up all the time I was taking off for doctor's visits. He conveniently forgot that I worked seven days a week and ten hours a day and actually delayed starting chemo until our computer program was functional. I even went back to work the day I passed out during the tonsil biopsy.

I won't go any further, as I want to keep as much negativity out of our book as possible.

My only advice is to put yourself first when your health hangs in the balance. If you are experiencing any pushback from your employer or coworkers, make sure you know your rights. Understand the company's policy, and make sure you look into the Family Medical Leave Act (FMLA) for your protection.

The good news for me was that shortly after this negative experience, I was able to begin a job at a school that valued me and worried about me. When I told my boss that I had leukemia, she thought of me, not the job. She immediately put hand sanitizers in the office and ordered me an air filter. I was always made to feel that my health mattered more than the job.

After finishing the sixth course of Rituximab, I was scheduled to take it on a maintenance basis. However, right before what would have been the second maintenance infusion, my blood work came back indicating a white cell count of .8. A normal count is in the range of 5 to 10.

Point 8 was not good.

Rituximab was discontinued, and I continued to take Mepron to ward off infections.

My experience with CLL has been that treatments work, and I am better as a result. Would I be in the same position today had I not been treated? I couldn't tell you, but I don't regret my decision.

Of course, I had doubts at the beginning. If CLL was not a big deal, why did I need toxic chemicals infused into my body? How would I react to chemo? How would all my efforts on damage control stand up to this new development? Would I need to take more time off from work? Would I be able to work? Would I lose my hair? Would I get sick?

The one question I never asked myself or even let come to the surface of my consciousness was whether chemo would keep me alive.

I am not sure if I was in such denial that I never considered the possibility that I could die, or that I had such unwavering faith in my medical team, including Eileen, that the thought never occurred to me. I never had any doubt about what we were doing — such was the depth of my faith in my team.

Before going for treatment, I had to schedule an appointment with the nurses to go over a few things.

Quite honestly, I missed most of the talk that followed after the first thing the nurse told me — from now on, I would have to flush the toilet twice when I peed, and I would have to use a condom during sex.

All I could think was *I'm fifty years old, I'm married, and I have to buy condoms*. I don't know what was worse, thinking about going to the drugstore to buy them, or the notion that I was now so toxic that having sex with me could be hazardous to my wife's health. It's not the kind of thing that triggers a steamy night of sex, is it?

When I received the news of my diagnosis, I was under no urgency to act. I was told that I could live as I always had. CLL is chronic, and there is no cure, but there is much debate as to whether treatment should ever be considered.

I read that there was little evidence to support the belief that the therapies available at that time would extend the life of a CLL patient. In fact, the harm to the immune system might well be more damaging than the disease.

How is anyone supposed to make a decision faced with such a difficult dilemma? You trust your doctor, that's how.

The most important thing that Eileen did for me (and for her, as it would later turn out) was to recommend that we meet with Dr. Avvento.

You know that old question about who you would choose to be in a foxhole with? Well, Dr. Avvento and Eileen would certainly be in there with me.

I know it may be hard to understand, but it got to the point that I actually looked forward to my appointments, and I always had to be prepared. Eileen would quiz me the night before: “What are you going to ask Dr. Avvento?”

I tried to stay current with the different therapies that were being tested so I could ask him about those, and I always made sure to tell him exactly how I felt.

On one occasion, I mentioned that I would be going down to Florida for the New York Yankees’ spring training. I brought it up to make sure I was okay to fly. You read how toxic airplane air is, and I just wanted to make sure I wasn’t putting myself at risk.

Anyway, he said it was fine for me to fly, but then we spoke about the Yankees for another fifteen minutes as he poked and prodded my lymph nodes and spleen.

That conversation proved once and for all that Dr. Avvento was not merely treating symptoms and blood counts but a human patient with a life. He was involved in my life more than my disease. It convinced me that this man would be the best one to ensure that my life continued.

So began my seventeen-year relationship with Dr. Louis Avvento and his team at Eastern Long Island Hematology and Oncology.

On that first visit in August of 2000, I was assured of a ten-year survival rate. Well, I am still here.

Over the years, Dr. Avvento has become much more than a clinician to my family and me. We talk as much about the Yankees, and especially the New York Rangers, as we do about CLL. His staff has been wonderful. Can you imagine feeling good about going to your oncologist? I have more angst getting a haircut.

Mirror, Mirror

I got a haircut on a Saturday afternoon — at a barbershop. That might not seem like anything to write about, but for a long time I avoided barbershops like the plague. This disinclination of mine to avoid barbershops began in the late 1960s. It was at that time, around 1969, that I started to grow my hair long in keeping with the times. Naturally, this abated whatever need I might have had for going to a barbershop in the first place. The side effect, in addition to longer hair, was that I now developed a phobia of making eye contact with my barber.

Tony the barber, not to be confused with the other Tony the barber, was a nice guy and was always kind to me whenever I passed by his shop or sat in his chair. He never cut me or tried to talk me out of those Mickey Mantle crew cuts. Now, I could hardly pass by his shop without a load of guilt. Here I was, this longhaired hippie (I was sure that's what he thought of me), taking money out of his pocket and food out of his family's mouth by never getting a haircut. Well, he probably never thought those things, but I felt bad, nonetheless.

So, this tonsorial phobia has continued ever since despite the fact that I have long ago moved away from the Bronx and Tony's barbershop. You might ask, "Surely you have gotten a haircut since 1969?" Of course, I have, but I have rarely gone to a barber. You see, my wife has indulged this phobia and has agreed to cut my hair for many if not most of the years we have been married...

until now. She has put her foot down, as well as her scissors and comb, and demanded that I regularly visit our local barber. Now a new phobia has developed.

Did you ever notice that barbershops have wall-to-wall mirrors? You can't help but see yourself, head suspended above that drop cloth they tuck you into. No matter where they spin you, there you are. It's frightening. It's even more frightening when I stare at the person looking back at me and realize it isn't me. It just couldn't be!

When I sat in Tony's chair, his mirrors only showed this kid talking about Mickey and Roger going back to back in yesterday's game. Now, this fat old bastard was sitting in my chair staring out at me and doing a great imitation of me, I might add, and I demand to know where he is keeping me prisoner!

I mean, it feels like I am in that *Star Trek* episode where Bones and Kirk age about ten years every minute, and by the end of the show, they are one hundred and eleven years old. There I am looking like I am a hundred and eleven explaining to the barber that my hair is thick in the back and on the sides, but watch up top, fella, as my crown is growing through, and if you use those funny scissors, I will be a modern St. Anthony.

So what do I do? Well, Saturday I closed my eyes for much of my haircut making believe that the barber was trimming my eyebrows. That's another thing! What's up with my eyebrows?

I am getting to feel like an American car that was made in the '70s. Any day now the wheels will fall off and my fenders will rust through. When did this happen?

Yesterday I had my monthly IVIG treatment. I have this scheduled on Fridays because it basically knocks me out for two days. So, there I am reading my iPad and listening to Jimmy Buffet on my iPhone, and this woman interrupts me to ask if I would like a massage or a Reiki treatment. It's a free service offered by the

Southampton Hospital Wellness Center. Now, I don't like anybody touching me. The massage thing is just something I wouldn't enjoy. I mean, it's supposed to be a relaxing thing, but if I got a massage, I would be as tense as a dried twig in a firestorm. So, what's the point?

However, I also have issues about saying no. I focused on the Reiki thing, as I know from Eileen's experience that she was able to get a virtual Reiki treatment. Her friend Pat was in New Jersey and phoned it in so to speak. So I'm thinking that this practitioner could be standing across the room and Reikiing me with no hands. Anyway, I agreed to have a Reiki treatment.

I told her to go to a few other people as I was just about into my Benadryl nap and didn't want to miss out on that, and I also secretly hoped that she would forget about me, but, alas, that was not to be, and she came over about a half hour later and nudged me. I had to stop listening to Jimmy Buffet, as that was not the proper mood music for a Reiki session. Fortunately, XM has a New Age station that was right up the Reiki alley, so I tuned in and turned on to the fabulous feeling of Reiki.

Now, as the foregoing has no doubt illustrated, I am a big skeptic. I only entered into this so as not to hurt this woman's feelings and, as I stated earlier, I hate to say no. The funny thing is I liked it.

I know there are other skeptics out there mocking me as you read this, but I think it worked. It was interesting to say the least. A few months ago, back in the summer, I hurt my right shoulder as I stumbled on the LIRR. (Howley, keep your snide remarks to yourself.) It has bothered me ever since. My Reiki provider started with my hands, and she advised me that there would not only be touching but compression. I am hyperventilating as I type this.

I really did try to relax and listen to the New Age channel, Spa. Again, no jokes please. So, she's working my fingers and hand, and then up my right arm and finally my right shoulder. I never said a word to her about my shoulder issue, but for some reason she stayed on that shoulder for a long time, longer than anywhere else. She then went to my feet and took my sneakers off (is this getting too racy for you?) and, again, it was very relaxing.

I go home after four hours in the treatment chair, and I am pretty knocked out as I usually am, but I don't have the usual aches and pains. I have been complaining about my leg for two weeks, and now it isn't bothering me anymore. I woke up Saturday and felt terrific. My shoulder doesn't hurt, my leg is better, and all in all I feel pretty good. I'm starting to feel really psyched about this Reiki thing. I was even able to kneel down at church. Hey, I even went to church for crying out loud! Okay, I started to lose it when the priest went on about something but that's a story for another book. I have to remember my experience and lose the inner tension that was the old Jimmy.

I am a believer. I have succumbed to Reiki.

One of the things that naturally happens when you are in a treatment setting for several hours is that you meet other patients. Some don't always respond to the treatment the way you do. I became friends with people who eventually passed away. One day they were getting treatment in the chair next to me. The next appointment, they were gone and someone else was in the chair, and the cycle continued. It's a reality check that you don't like to dwell on, but it is right there in front of you nonetheless.

Having cancer makes you learn not to take anything or anyone for granted. Family and friends have been with me through this entire journey. The same group was there for Eileen and me when Eileen was going through her journey. Sometimes I wonder, why us? But then I look around and realize that I have nothing to complain about. On the contrary, I have so much to be grateful for. We have been blessed with so many people that have cared for us. Our circle of friends has expanded at the time of life when it usually recedes. To complain about what life has presented would seem silly.

Yankee Baseball Therapy

I have been a Yankee fan practically my entire life. My earliest recollection was that on my sixth birthday, my Uncle Al gave me a Yankee hat, this wasn't just another store-bought Yankee hat.

In 1956, Major League Baseball had not discovered marketing. You couldn't go to a store and pick out a hat or a shirt or a jersey with the name of your favorite team or player emblazoned on the front. You might be able to purchase a blue cap with the felt letters NY ironed on the crown, but you certainly couldn't get an official New York Yankees hat — unless you knew Uncle Al.

Uncle Al was married to my Aunt Catherine, and he just might have been the sweetest person in the world. I always describe him as Stanley to my father's Ollie. When the two of them got together, it was like being on the set of a Laurel and Hardy movie.

My favorite story about them occurred at Uncle Al and Aunt Catherine's house in Rosendale, New York. In those days, we called it "up the country," and it seemed so far away from the Bronx. Anyway, Uncle Al always had a project going. For example, he had a somewhat weathered (being kind here) Ford "woody" station wagon circa 1935. In addition to being just a little rough around the edges, it lacked a roof, a minor hurdle to overcome for Uncle Al.

He saw this car at an auction, and knowing a bargain when he saw one, Uncle Al purchased the roofless woody and made plans for the following week. When the next Saturday arrived, Uncle Al went to another auction and purchased a roof.

Sadly, this roof was designed for a Chevy and was no match for his Ford.

Well, Uncle Al was a driver for Railway Express Agency, which at the time was akin to United Parcel Service or FedEx. As luck would have it, Yankee Stadium was on my Uncle Al's route. He would, during the course of the day, make a trip or two into the Yankee clubhouse delivering all sorts of packages for the team. Players knew him and gave him a nod or a hello, and sometimes he talked with them.

On more than one occasion, he had gotten us a few baseballs that had been used for batting practice, and we always loved when he came to visit loaded up with some New York Yankee treasure.

As early as 1956, I had been thoroughly indoctrinated by my father and brother Mike to be a Yankee fan and, in particular, a Mickey Mantle fan. Knowing this, my uncle approached Mickey Mantle and asked him to sign a hat for his little nephew. Mickey did so, and Uncle Al gave it to me on June 23, 1956.

It should be noted that this was a real New York Yankee hat with the interlocking NY stitched on the crown. You wouldn't see a hat like this for sale for quite a while, and only when sports leagues recognized they had an opportunity to make a lot of money by selling official, licensed team merchandise.

1956 was an exceptional year in Mickey Mantle lore. He had won the triple crown in one of the best years a baseball player could have. A hat signed by Mickey in 1956 is worth a fortune.

Sadly, nothing was known about memorabilia in 1956, and the hat that my uncle so thoughtfully gave to me for my sixth birthday was worn by me every spring and summer day until I was a teenager, and it died a natural death due to regular wear and tear. It disintegrated on my head.

So began my love affair with the Yankees.

I passed along the Yankee gene to my three children and would often take them to Yankee games. We saw some memorable games over the years, and in 2002, the year after I finished chemo, I purchased a mini-season ticket plan for every Saturday game in Yankee Stadium.

Initially, Bryan and I went to the games, as Sean and Jeannine had summer jobs, but now and then they joined us. It just so happened that during this time, from the day I received my diagnosis (and for quite a few years before) until the present day, the Yankees have had tremendous success.

We have seen tremendous players and have had a great time going to games. I do not doubt that purchasing this season ticket plan was part of my therapy for dealing with cancer. Going to games with my kids and friends was as important an affirmation of living the good life as a boy from the Bronx could make.

Going to these games was so much more than merely watching the Yankees play baseball. In fact, we often spent more time talking than watching. As my children got older, going to these games gave us the opportunity to grow in our relationship. Always the teacher, I used these opportunities to instruct and advise.

Of course, one of the topics I always included was never to have a commute like mine. On one occasion, Sean and I were at the game, and he assured me that I didn't have to worry; he would never commute as I had done. I confessed to him that my being away from home so much had been detrimental to him and Jeannine and Bryan.

"I was never there," I said.

He replied, "What are you talking about? You were always there."

When Sean said that, I was brought back to another conversation when he was about eight or nine. I had asked him if his friends went to baseball games or football games, and he said they didn't. I asked why not.

He answered, "Because they don't have a dad like you."

The Joke's On Me

Shortly after I was diagnosed, I experienced a form of euphoria. Trust me, I was not ecstatic to hear that I had CLL, but I felt a certain amount of liberation in realizing that, compared to cancer, job hassles and mortgage payments were no longer major concerns.

In fact, those concerns were in the way-way back of my consciousness.

I also used humor to fight the disease.

Eileen was probably thinking that this was all part of my denial strategy. I made jokes and tried to show my family that I was fine. Not everyone appreciated my humor, of course. I learned a few years later that some of my witticisms sent my daughter, Jeannine, crying to her mother.

Another one of my ploys was to feign fatigue and weakness, and ask her to "get Daddy a beer" or do some other task like empty the dishwasher or fold the laundry, all while wearing a pained expression to emphasize my misery.

I thought I was being funny, but I was the only one who laughed. I have found that I am often my best audience, and, in truth, the only one who appreciates some of my poorer attempts at humor.

I guess I was able to do this because I really didn't feel sick. Believe me, I am no martyr, and I wouldn't have put on a brave front if I had not felt well. Even when I was getting chemo, I felt okay. I had fatigue, and when I got home from work, I crashed for the evening, but I got up the next day and drove sixty miles to work. Then I left work and drove sixty, actually seventy miles to the next day's chemo, and so on for the entire week of chemotherapy.

I was fortunate because I had good support systems at home and at work. My staff was spectacular; the higher ups also had their moments.

I guess the one moment of despair occurred toward the third or fourth cycle of chemo. Because I had to leave the office early to get to my oncologist's office for treatment, I was not always around for meetings. I began to feel that I was out of the loop. Worse, it felt like I was intentionally being left out of the loop.

On one occasion, a person from another office went to my Associate Director to ask a question. I felt that as the Director I should have been consulted. I felt overlooked and disrespected. So, I did a stupid thing and wrote an email to this woman with the subject matter PROTOCOL—yes, in all caps in case she didn't get the message.

I proceeded to state that if she needed information, she should start with me. I later learned that she showed the email to one of her colleagues who also knew me as a friend.

She asked, appropriately, "What's up Jim Newell's ass?"

My friend told her that there must be something wrong, as I am not usually like that. She let it go.

Well, I felt like a schmo. I had never behaved like that in the workplace. I may have thought things and gotten myself worked up at times, but I never acted on those feelings.

This episode made me realize that I was being affected by CLL and the chemo. I realized that I was not Superman, and I was sick.

It took me a long time to repair the damage that I had caused. Well, I guess I was making more of it than the woman I had accused of not following protocol. Anyway, I was awkward with her, and it was important that we work well together.

I didn't know what to say, and soon that became painfully obvious. We were trying to schedule a meeting, and I announced that I couldn't make the date suggested because it conflicted with my next chemotherapy treatment.

As soon as I said it, I could see that we were friends again. In fact, a few weeks later, I talked to her about the email, and she laughed and told me what she had asked my friend.

I learned that allowing myself to get depressed and all worked up did not help me. I know some might say that I was entitled to feel that way, and I certainly can empathize with anyone who does get depressed during treatment or at any time dealing with CLL or any type of cancer. For me, however, I needed to stay positive.

I began to view my chemotherapy sessions as an escape from the drudgery of the world of financial aid. I read books and listened to music on my Nano iPod that my kids gave me loaded with my favorite songs.

A major reason I was able to stay positive was because the chemo was working. My lymph nodes shrank significantly. My spleen reduced in size. My white blood cell counts went down, and my platelets went up. My doctor was happy, and assured me that I was on the mend.

The one complaint I did have was that I was gaining weight. This was odd to me. I had always heard stories about cancer patients losing so much weight. When I brought this up, my doctor said that he was not worried about my weight gain. I guess when all is said and done, a little extra girth is a modest price to pay for better health.

The off weeks, when I was not being treated, were relatively normal. By the time Monday came, I was back to working full days and even into the evening. I would get home around 7:30 p.m. and have a normal evening of dinner, a little TV, and getting ready for the next day.

As I mentioned, I had great support systems. My family was there every step of the way. Sean was away at Fordham, and I was worried about how he was dealing with things, so we made an effort to go see him every now and then.

Jeannine and Bryan were still living at home, and they could see what I was going through, but I don't think they saw anything alarming.

Eileen was a rock, or so it appeared.

One of the things I only learned when she was dealing with breast cancer nearly ten years later was that being a caregiver was not that easy. In fact, I felt a little ashamed considering how I made such a big deal over my illness. When she saw how I was not coping well with her illness, she let me in on a little secret. She hadn't always coped well with mine either. The difference is she never let me see her not coping. I was not that considerate. Well, I have a bad poker face, and I tend to cry a lot.

Looking back, I have to laugh at myself.

There I was trying to put a positive spin on things, making jokes and being silly, completely unaware that Eileen was not buying it for a second. She said I was in denial, and maybe I was. I don't know. I do know that dwelling on the disease and treatment and stressing out at work didn't do me any good or anyone close to me, for that matter.

Laughter may not be the best medicine, but it does help us heal, and genuine humor helps us cope with what could be an otherwise very dark journey.

My childhood friends would check in on me, and while I know they were concerned, we always managed a good laugh on those occasions when we met for a cocktail or spoke on the phone.

You have to laugh.

I started laughing at my first visit to the oncologist when a nurse practitioner had to perform a bone marrow biopsy. I mean, when you see the size of that needle, and she tells you she is going to stick it in your hip so pull your pants down, you just start to giggle.

Right after that torture session, I took Bryan to play baseball.

Bryan was a good hitter, and I would pitch to him. Earlier that summer he hit a line drive that I caught right in the thigh. My glove didn't catch it; my thigh did. I had a massive black-and-blue on that thigh for a month. So there I was, pitching to him, still bleeding a little from the biopsy, and all I could think about was getting hit by a line drive. Thankfully, he only hit long fly balls that day.

When I was newly married and visited my parents on Leland Avenue in the Bronx, my mother always offered me a twenty-dollar bill, and of course, I always thanked her. One time she said, "You don't mind me still giving you money, do you?" I said,

"No Mom, you have to let other people do good things for you sometimes." I think she liked that response.

I tried to keep that in mind when I was going through chemo.

Although I was able to drive myself to and from my sessions, very often my brother Johnny or brother-in-law Jimmy drove me. It gave them an opportunity to do something for me, and it certainly allowed me to relax and enjoy their company.

It would be a terrible disease indeed if it did not bring families together.

Playing With Trains And Being In Control

When I tell people how long my commute is, they are stunned and amazed that it literally takes me two hours to get to work. Sometimes they look at me as if I am nuts. That is why I don't tell them it is two hours each way.

Actually, the *real* reason I don't tell them is because it's closer to three hours each way.

Why then would someone who spends nearly thirty hours a week on some kind of railway want to spend his leisure time playing with trains? Maybe I am nuts?

I was on my way home from a conference in San Diego when I started thinking. Flying can be relaxing unless you are in front of annoying people who constantly kick your seat or slam the tray at your back. Thank God for noise reduction headphones. Anyway, I was relaxed and had a long flight ahead of me, so I let my mind wander as I listened to my favorite music.

One of the conference sessions dealt with the choices students make. I realized there was a lot going on with the choices I was making relative to playing with Lionel trains, so I decided to talk to Eileen about this, and she observed that I wanted to return to my carefree childhood years.

That makes sense. I am playing with trains that were either produced in the late Forties or in the Fifties. They were given to me by my parents when I was not yet a teenager. I was indoctrinated in the love of trains by my brother Mike, and Lionel trains were a passion that we continued to share well into adulthood.

But I think my love of Lionel trains is more than mere nostalgia. I think it's about control.

You see, if we want to be honest about it, the 1940s (I hear!) were not always pleasant. Our parents had World War II to worry about, not to mention the whiplash caused by the Great Depression of the Thirties. It wasn't always the Andrews Sisters jitterbugging and Bing Crosby crooning. Life was hard.

The Fifties were no bargain either. No sooner had people gotten used to the post-war peace than Korea exploded and more Americans were killed. The post-war economic boom was not equally distributed to all, and people started to take note that not all Americans were treated equally. The H Bomb made us hide under our desks in practice drills that would've been useless had a bomb really been dropped, and fall-out shelters were built in peoples' back yards or, as on Leland Avenue, in the basements of apartment buildings. Yet, we called this a happy time.

To be fair, hindsight might be 20/20, but we don't always see those frightening things when we look in the rearview mirror. They seem to get filtered out, and we tend to focus only on the fun things. I think this is a survival mechanism. No sense dwelling on the pain of life.

So, when I immerse myself in my train collection, I do not think I am trying to return to the days of my youth. I think I want to return to a time when I was in control. Of course, I was never

ever in control, so there is no time to which I can return, but I can build that time on a 4 x 8 sheet of plywood.

On this sheet of wood, I can construct a New York City — complete with the Empire State Building, the Chrysler Building, and even the Ed Sullivan Theater — where there is no crime, and the trains run on time. On my subway line there are no muggers and no need for stop-and-frisk laws, and of course, there are no newspapers or irritating talking heads.

In my Yankee Stadium, there is no talk of steroids or AROD, and the Red Sox continue to lose. The soundtrack of my Yankee Stadium continues to play Sinatra singing "New York, New York," and "Enter Sandman" will always play at the appropriate time of day.

Economically speaking, America is still a manufacturing country in my world as coal is delivered to factories that churn out automobiles that need to be delivered, and the dairy and cattle industries continue to thrive. While I have a nuclear reactor, it is safe, and even the nuclear waste that I transport is securely housed in leak-proof containers.

The Cold War persists, but we are protected by minuteman cars and missile launchers. We have not yet reached the moon in my reconstructed world, but our space program is thriving.

More important to my present day concerns, passenger service on my train line is always on time, and no one ever mentions Mussolini on my trains. We do get snow from time to time, but it never causes a delay, and the only time we shut down service is when it is time for all of us to go to bed.

The ZW transformer is all I ever need to keep things running. If only the real world were so easily controlled.

I have no doubt that continuing to enjoy model railroading as my brother Mike and I always did has helped me with Mike's loss. I feel his presence when I play with the trains. Like any hobby, playing with trains allows me to escape, if only for a few minutes, the harsh realities of a life that is often complicated with treatments and weight gain and recalcitrant hair.

Jimmy Newell's Dream

One of the things that for the most part has kept me well grounded is remembering my mother and father, and trying to imagine how they would react to my cancer diagnosis, and wondering what advice they would give. I wish they had been blessed with longevity and were still with us today.

Thinking of my parents reminds me of a dream I had during my cancer treatments, but first a little background information.

I had made it through that first year of CLL pretty well, all things considered. I got through the six courses of chemo. I survived telling my children and didn't reveal to them just how scared I really was. Now, as we approached spring and the onset of a new baseball season, I felt like I was getting back to normal.

Bryan would be graduating from elementary school in June, and we were planning a two-week vacation to Disney beginning the day after he graduated. That buoyed my spirits better than any medication could possibly have done.

Before Disney and even before opening day of the new baseball season, there was St. Patrick's Day.

St. Patrick's Day has always been more than just an opportunity to drink cheap, green beer. Most of my favorite memories of the Irish holiday actually have nothing at all to do with drinking. The association of alcohol with being Irish was something my mother always hated despite the fact that she enjoyed a drink or two on occasion.

For her, St. Patrick's Day was first and foremost a religious holiday. We were always off from school because we attended Catholic school, but she made sure we went to Mass. Despite it falling during Lent, we were never strictly held accountable to our Lenten sacrifices, and thus we imbibed and ingested all sorts of holiday treats, specifically Irish soda bread with just enough butter, marmalade, and raspberry preserves. I guess the sugar rush substituted for the alcohol.

Back then I wasn't much for corned beef, but my father was, and Momma made sure he had his cabbage to go with it.

No St. Patrick's Day was complete without getting a packet of shamrocks from my Aunt Katie in Sligo and watching Jack, AKA Captain Jack McCarthy host the NYC parade. Back then there were no debates about who could march and who couldn't, and as long as Jack narrated the festivities with a rich, faux brogue, we were all happy. It's funny how simple things are preserved in such strong memories.

Often on St. Patrick's Day, I think of those loved ones who are no longer with me. I am sure I am not alone in that regard. My brother Johnny and I often met for dinner, and one of his favorite topics was asking the question, "Wouldn't it be nice if all the people we have lost could come back one day a year, just to talk?"

So here I am sitting in front of my fireplace on St. Patrick's Day. I confess I have a wee dram of the crayture, a little Johnny Jameson's best. It helps set the mood.

The Irish soda bread, my mother's recipe, is just out of the oven. The smell is fantastic; you can taste it, can't you? I cut off the heel, as it's my favorite piece, and the one always saved for me by Lizzie McHugh AKA Momma. As I wash down the first bite with a little taste of whiskey, I gaze at the fire and watch the swirls of smoke wafting up the chimney.

But then, just as the smoke finds its way skyward, another shape takes its place.

She looks as I remember her best. Her hair is freshly coiffed by Chuck, her grandson, who she often referred to as Chip. Her glasses are on, and the smile that lit up the Crossroads in Sligo and all of Leland Avenue in the Bronx was more intoxicating than anything the Jamesons ever distilled.

At times like this, it does no good to ask how or why. You just have to accept the blessing and enjoy the moment.

We started talking like it had only been a week since our last conversation rather than eighteen years. I told her we all call her Nana now, as we often talk about her to the kids and the others who did not have the joy to know her. She was fine with that; hearing a fifty-year-old man call her Momma was more than she could handle. But she didn't see me as a middle-aged man, but rather as the thirty-two-year-old I was when she left.

Nana asked about Eileen and the kids. She always laughed about the grandchildren and Eileen, and my contribution received the same loving smile and laughter. She seemed to know all the stories about them before I finished telling them. She even told her own stories about them, things I didn't know. The only thing that made her feel bad was knowing how much they missed not knowing her.

We continued talking, and eventually, I asked about Pop. "Oh, he's coming," she said with certainty. "You can ask him yourself."

You would think that witnessing such a phenomenon would have inspired me to ask countless questions. You'd be right. However, I never got the chance to ask one question. Nana and Pop did all the talking.

Pop started out by shaking his head in amazement that I was still commuting all that way into the city. He said, "You know, Jimmy, I worked hard all my life, since I was thirteen, but watching you and all that you do, well, all I can say is you make me very proud."

Nana chimed in. "Now, Daddy Dear, he wouldn't have been able to write that book had he not had all that time to do nothing but read and write." She was referring to my first book, a memoir of my childhood and young adult years called *A Bronx Boy's Tale*.

I was stunned at what Pop said and that Nana knew of my book.

"You know about the book?" I asked.

"Yes, Luv, who wouldn't know about the book? That's all you seem to talk about lately."

I don't know how, but as she said that, her smile got even bigger and more radiant, and then we all had a great laugh at the expense of my humanity and hubris.

She then went on to say that while she liked the book, "It would have been better had you not resorted to so many examples of pagan language."

I said, "Mom, for crying out loud, I used the F-word once!"

"Sure, that's not the only example of Satan's speech."

Pop then talked about all the baseball games that I took the kids to over the years. Again, that was something that made him proud. It also made him a little bit guilty, I think, as he lamented that he should have taken me to see Mickey Mantle more often.

I then began to come to my senses and asked about Michael, and I was told he was grand. When I asked where he was and why he wasn't here to talk with me right now like they were doing, I was told that I wasn't on everyone's top of the list, but he would come to visit me some day.

"Well, don't you want to know about Maureen and Barbara and Johnny?" I asked.

"Luv, I know it's hard to understand, so I won't even attempt to explain, but we are with them too now. Like you, they just have to turn around and start talking."

I could go on, but right now, I just want to continue my St. Patrick's Day visit.

Sliante.

Dreams or visions can often serve therapeutic purposes. For me, St. Patrick's Day 2001 was my last course of therapy that would keep me in good health for quite a few years.

Just Rolling Along When All Of A Sudden

The one thing I have learned is that when it comes to cancer, you are always in the woods.

There may be extended periods of remission or indolence, but you are only one doctor's appointment from the reality of your disease.

In the spring of 2016, what I thought to be unrelated to CLL turned out to be something that CLL patients often develop. I thought I had a sebaceous cyst on my head. It was a small pimple-sized cyst for a week or so, and then it quickly erupted into a much bigger cyst.

I made an appointment with a dermatologist to see what could be done to alleviate this growth. A biopsy was performed, and even before the results were determined, I was advised that it was a squamous carcinoma.

Carcinoma caught my attention.

I was reassured that it was serious enough to respect but not to worry about, and an appointment for MOHS surgery (a type of microscopic skin surgery named after its inventor, Fredrick Mohs, MD) was made.

That surgery went really well. My dermatologist was terrific, and has been added to my medical team. But my summer continued to offer surprises.

I had been fighting a cold all summer. My white blood cell counts were elevated, and I had a feeling I would be going through another round of treatment soon.

In fact, my hematologist/oncologist Dr. Louis Avvento and I had talked about it the previous year, but he felt that I could continue without treatment. A year can make a big difference in cancer treatment, and now it was time.

I started daily doses of Ibrutinib in September 2016. So far, I have had great results. My white cell count has gone down. My lymph nodes and spleen have reduced in size, and I generally feel better. I no longer seem congested.

Eileen and I were in the midst of selling our house and moving to Florida during this time. As luck would have it, I had another episode with a cyst. This time it was a sebaceous cyst, but on my chest, which required that it be drained.

I resumed the Ibrutinib a few days after the procedure, but I had a bleeding issue, so I discontinued after one dose.

I waited another week but had the same result.

Dr. Avvento ordered a sonogram, which revealed a lot of fluid that was not going away on its own. Surgery was necessary.

Again, I was off Ibrutinib, and this time it would be for several weeks.

As if we didn't have enough stress in our lives, Eileen and I were due to move on January 16, 2017, and my surgery was set for January 9.

We had to pack up and get out of the house in one week. Fortunately, our kids, in-laws, and friends helped us, as they have done so many times.

In less than six months, we had discovered a new place to call home over a thousand miles away from our family and friends. We sold our dream house where we had lived for thirty-three years and raised our kids, and were awaiting the completion of our new house in Bradenton, Florida.

The stitches from my surgery had yet to be removed after we were settled in Florida. What a whirlwind!

At this point, I have to add another story about Pop.

In 1976, right before Eileen and I were to be married, my mother and father moved out of their apartment in the Bronx and into a beautiful garden apartment in Atlantic Highlands, New Jersey, where my sister Maureen and her family lived. It was a gorgeous apartment.

Except, my father hated it.

In less than a month, he had convinced my mother to move back to the Bronx. She acquiesced because she was worried about his mental well-being. He moped around all day long, and she had to do something.

I add this story because I am, after all, my father's son.

So much change in such a short time was not easy for me. I missed my kids badly. I missed their dogs—maybe even more!

Even though I was in paradise, it took some time to get used to being so far away from everyone who mattered to me.

Then, a little more than two months after we left East Quogue, my brother Johnny died. I was devastated. He was my big brother. He was always someone I tried to live up to. He was in the Marines during the Korean War when I was two, and I remember running down the street and jumping into his waiting arms when he came home.

We used to meet for dinner once a month, and even though we talked on the phone every day after I moved to Florida, I always felt I'd abandoned him.

With all of this emotion coming at me, I recovered from the surgery and resumed my Ibrutinib regimen.

I don't take anything for granted, and try to enjoy retirement in Florida. You have to stay positive and make every moment a special one because you are alive to talk and laugh with your family and friends, to see the sun rise and set, to walk on the beach, to smell the rain, and even to watch the grass grow, which is literally possible during rainy Florida summers.

Eileen Reflects On Jimmy's Diagnosis

I am married to a very generous, loving man. Throughout his life, he knew he wanted to write. So he started to write a book about twenty years ago, and during the living of our life, he put the book writing aside. He was working full time, going to law school, and raising his family — no time to write. Eventually, after I sent him a link to a publishing site, he was inspired to continue with his book. I always believed that he felt compelled to leave his children a legacy from his childhood, and so *A Bronx Boy's Tale* was published in 2013.

When I was forty-six, I noticed something about my husband. He was tired a lot, and I was doing a lot of the chores. Because of his stressful job, long workdays, and the ridiculous commute, it seemed reasonable that he would be tired. I never thought there was anything wrong with him.

But then I noticed a change. He seemed to be feeling achy, and he exhibited flu-like symptoms most of the time. Of course, he seemed unaware of this while it was happening, and continued to be oblivious to what I was seeing.

I asked him to go to the doctor for a checkup. He was fifty, and it was about time he had a tune-up. I never dreamt there was anything seriously wrong with Jimmy.

The two of us were just returning to work, having been on vacation for a week. I was always a little stressed out when I returned to work after a vacation, but little did I know what was in store for me that day.

Jimmy called me at work early in the day and told me the doctor had just called him with the lab results from his physical. He was diagnosed with CLL.

I was not really prepared for this diagnosis. I suspected that something was wrong, but I didn't have cancer in mind.

I'd been a nurse for more than twenty-five years, and I found it very hard to separate the clinician from the concerned wife. Seeing Jimmy put up a brave front did nothing to assuage my fears.

While Jimmy was surfing the internet, I immediately went into crisis management mode. I reached out to his primary care physician who performed the physical. Then, my worst fears confirmed, I called a hematologist/oncologist that I had known for several years and set the rest of the week in motion.

Thank God I had such great friends at work who were a constant source of support for Jimmy and me.

Later that evening when Jimmy got home from work, I could tell he was concerned, but he didn't seem too worried. He was either being brave or in denial. To this day, I am not sure which. All he kept repeating was that he didn't feel sick.

The next day we met with Dr. Louis Avvento, the hematologist/oncologist. He was very reassuring and had a positive attitude. At this first meeting, we were told about the staging of leukemia. This is where I learned that Jimmy was hearing what he wanted to hear.

We learned that Jimmy was in stage four. Now, Jimmy still believes he heard that it was stage four using an eight-stage system that he read about on the internet. It wasn't. It was stage four using the standard four-stage system, which meant that Jimmy was in trouble.

Side note: It's important to know about the staging of your cancer because that's how they determine the treatment options. Notice I said options. You will get to look at the options and determine with your team which one will work best for your cancer cells. To get the right staging, you need the tissue and the pathologist. Ask for a copy of your reports and start to build the story of your own journey. Make this a habit.

Jimmy was not anemic, but he did have enlarged lymph nodes and an enlarged spleen, and although his white count was high, it wasn't so high that it required immediate treatment. Dr. Avvento anticipated that he would not treat at this time, but when he saw the results of the biopsy, he decided that treatment was in order.

I put up a brave front and never let down my guard in front of Jimmy. It was years later, when facing my own battle with cancer, that I let him in on my little secret. There were times during his treatment when I was a complete mess.

Jimmy started chemo in October 2000 and completed the treatment in February. He seemed better. In only a few short months after his last chemo session, he was playing racquetball a couple of nights a week with our son Bryan.

He began going to Yankee games, and, while the words cure or remission were not used, I could tell that he had turned the corner on CLL.

The thing I have learned about CLL is that you can never know for sure where it is heading. Even though Jimmy's CLL was indolent, it could turn into a non-Hodgkin's form of lymphoma. Richter's Transformation or Richter's Syndrome frightened me and was always on my mind anytime Jimmy went to see Dr. Avvento.

One day I was in the basement worrying over his disease, and I realized that my fear was holding me back. I was spending so much time worrying about what *could* happen that I was not living. I was putting things on hold. This was a defining moment for me. I spoke to Jimmy about this and mentioned we needed to expand our house. To me, this was powerfully symbolic. It meant that we had a future filled with family, friends, and good times. Secretly, I thought if he did get sicker, he would have a beautiful room to be in.

As I think back on everything that cancer has put us through together, I realize that we've coped as best we could, moment by moment, because there's nothing else you can do. But I've also learned that you don't go through something like this as a family without some turmoil.

When Jimmy was diagnosed with cancer, all I could think about was my mother. My father died when I was a year old. He left my mother with five children to raise and a house to pay for.

My mother worked two jobs and was gone until well into the evening. My older brother Patrick and my sister Mary were my surrogate parents.

I became frightened that I would be facing a life of hardship, just like my mother had endured.

I decided to change my job and go back to school after thirty years to earn my Bachelor of Science in Nursing. I took classes online so that I could do most of my schoolwork at home.

Looking back at that time, I am amazed at how I met that challenge. I didn't know how to use a computer, but I learned. I wanted to get my degree so that if something happened to Jimmy, and I should become the sole breadwinner, my children would still be able to have a good life.

I worked full-time in the day and was a full-time student at night. There wasn't much living going on. I was very focused on schoolwork, but it was worth it. I graduated and attained my BSN in nursing.

I was thrilled with my accomplishment and with the support I got from family and friends to finish school.

Little did I know that it was nothing like the support I would get five years later when it was my turn to be the cancer patient.

Not The Fireworks We Expected

My mother had to raise a family on her own and worked two jobs to do so. She never had time to take a day off or to call in sick when she was not feeling well. She was of the generation some refer to as the greatest, but she only saw herself as a working mother. She did what she had to do. There was no other choice.

So, when she got sick, you knew she was *really* sick, and it was serious. I guess I am my mother's daughter, because that's how it was with me. I got sick suddenly, and it was serious.

Jimmy and I were just rebounding from his diagnosis and treatments and settling into the groove of enjoying life again. We had just completed the addition to our home in East Quogue when we had to face the prospect of cancer once again.

It felt like the home we had worked so hard to create was under siege. We were being attacked by that damn, dreaded disease once again. It felt like I could never get away from cancer. No matter where I was in life, it was lurking around the next corner waiting to jump out and say, "Gotcha!"

First, it was my father, who I never got a chance to know because leukemia took him when I was an infant. Then my brother Patrick lost his battle to Hodgkin's disease shortly after Jimmy and I were married.

My mother lost her battle with cancer eight years later.

Then, instead of having a fiftieth birthday party for Jimmy, we had to schedule chemo treatments. What next?

Breast cancer, that's what!

I found out a day before Bryan was leaving for London, right before the Fourth of July weekend, but I didn't tell anyone until after the weekend.

It wasn't enough that I knew what I was in for: a radical mastectomy, harsh chemo, losing my hair, radiation treatments. On top of all of this, I had to prepare Jimmy. God help me.

Don't get me wrong. I knew Jimmy would be okay. He had gone through so much already fighting his leukemia. He had been a good patient from the beginning, and as a longtime nurse, I knew the difference between a bad patient and a good patient. He was always more worried about us than himself, but the roles would be reversed now. He would be the caregiver, and I would be the patient.

I saw how Jimmy was when my brother Patrick got sick, and then when his brother Michael lost his battle and passed away. Jimmy persevered through it all, but it took a lot out of him. I had always wondered whether Michael's passing and Jimmy's illness were related. Sometimes it seemed like a distinct possibility. But now I had a new concern.

How was Jimmy going to react to my cancer?

I made up my mind that I was not going to sugarcoat it. I was going to be honest. My prognosis was questionable because the cancer cells had spread into my lymph system. Jimmy needed to know that, and I needed him to be strong. If it meant that I had to be brutally honest, then so be it.

The evening I broke the news to him, I could see that he would need time to adjust to this new normal. He understood what I said, but it really didn't hit him. I knew that would happen when our children were there. I just had to wait a few days.

I was going to have surgery in a matter of weeks followed by chemo, and then life as we knew it would never be the same.

Before the kids came out that weekend, we talked, and I prepared him for what was going to happen.

Jimmy always loved my breasts, but when I told him about the surgery, he only said, "I fell in love with your eyes, not your breasts."

I knew then that he would be okay, but he still had to get there.

The weekend came and the kids were coming out to visit. Our friends Vinnie and Maryanne were also coming out, and my sister Mary and my brother Jimmy were too.

I scheduled an appointment with my surgeon for Monday, and the weekend would serve as a good distraction. There was a music festival on the North Fork of Long Island, and a typical Saturday night mixed grill would be just what the doctor ordered — for now.

I went out to our local farmer's market only to return to a locked door that was opened by a crying sixty-year-old. Jimmy had been alone in the house listening to his beloved Jimmy Buffet, and he had lost it. He'd had a complete meltdown.

"Come Monday" on the radio broke through Jimmy's defensive shell, and the reality of what we were facing had its impact.

Once I was able to calm him down and the kids made their way in, he was able to help plan the day. Then Vinnie and Maryanne came in.

Vinnie had been our parish priest when we were kids in the Bronx at Blessed Sacrament and, although no longer a priest, no one made us feel more spiritual than Vinnie.

He wanted to pray with us as a family, and we certainly needed to pray. We all sat in our living room and closed our eyes, as Vinnie suggested. Well, I cheated.

I was worried about Jimmy. He had calmed down from his earlier meltdown, but I knew he was doing his best to hold it together. A few minutes into the prayer, I could see I was right to keep an eye on him.

Jimmy was heaving up and down, not making a sound but shaking with grief and doing his best not to bawl out loud. I went over to him and tried to console him.

That made him laugh.

He said, "Here you are facing this terrible thing, and all you can do is worry about me."

I knew what he was going through because I had gone through the exact same thing when he was diagnosed. Worrying about someone else is always harder than worrying about yourself.

Eileen's Treatment Begins

To start the treatment, there are a series of questions. Where? Who? What? The things you take for granted are now in front of you as you ponder the best place, the best surgeon, and which procedure/treatment plan is right for you. This is the most important decision you will make for your survival, and my ultimate decision surprised me as well as many others in my life. I stayed local, and it was the best decision. For breast cancer, the treatment regimen is pretty well standardized. Not all cancers are like this, so give your treatment options your full attention. You want no regrets as you navigate this journey.

First I had a bilateral mastectomy, a twelve-hour surgery that required an overnight stay in the hospital. Shortly after my surgery, I started chemotherapy. You need to be in good physical condition before you start. Ask your doctor and nurses what this means for you. One of the important things is to see a dentist, because you want to ensure there are no infections looming in your teeth and gums.

The first day of treatment, bring a close friend who can be a support for you. I avoided my family members because I knew it would be hard on them. Bring a distraction with you. Read up on what your role is as a chemo patient. In knowing your role, you are helping yourself while your doctors and healthcare team are helping you.

One of the things that always annoyed me was when people, with good intentions, told tales of friends or family who had breast cancer, and all were alive and well, and they got through everything in a breeze. I learned my cancer cells are mine alone, because all our cells are unique to us as individuals. Once I realized that, I dismissed "those" stories when things weren't so easy for me.

Then, there are those well-intentioned good wishers who tell you that you look terrific.

I have no hair, I have no breasts, and I look terrific???

It was all I could do to keep from saying, "Fuck you!"

I began a regimen of Adriamycin, often referred to as the Red Devil. There's nothing good I can write about this chemotherapy. I am convinced that it almost killed me.

I don't know how many cycles of chemo I had received when I found myself in the emergency room. My first visit was due to an elevated temperature and chills. I had sores in my mouth and couldn't get fluids down. I was in bed more than out of bed. Something was not right. My son was home and had to take me. Once there I had fluids intravenously, and I felt much better. They did the cursory tests, but all were negative because I was already on antibiotics. I was happy to go home. Lesson learned: pay attention to how you feel and act on it immediately.

Shortly after that illness, I woke up one morning not feeling well at all. At one point, I lost all sense of balance and was convinced that I had gone head over heels in my bed.

I made my way to the bathroom and could not get off the toilet. The side effects of chemo were kicking in. Vomiting and diarrhea were non-stop. I didn't think I could get out of the bathroom, and I felt myself slipping into unconsciousness. It wasn't getting any better. Jimmy was with me, and I told him to call for an ambulance, but he didn't want to. He said, "I can take you — you don't need an ambulance."

It wasn't that he didn't want to help me or provide the care I needed. I think he knew I was slipping away, and calling an ambulance was not happening on his watch.

The episode passed, and Jimmy drove me to the hospital where I was admitted.

As remarkable as modern medicine is, there are times when all the physicians can do is shake their heads and speculate. It might have been and most probably was meningitis. I stayed in the hospital for a few days, and my chemo was delayed a month so I could regain my strength.

Jimmy has already mentioned how he dealt with his chemo. I was not as fortunate as he, and it was so very hard for me to get through it. I don't know if I could do that again.

In my daily life, I had to work on living without the things I normally had. The most obvious of those were my breasts. But the most unexpected things I lost, or that were impaired, were my hearing, my balance, my ability to feel my toes, and my memory.

I had always loved relying on my memory because memories bring joy, confidence, a little sadness, but most importantly, memory is something we heavily rely on to live our life. Now I wasn't so confident in this skill I had taken for granted. I was living in a fog. I relied on others for the simple things I had managed all my life. Chemo brain is real. It has long-lasting effects for some people. Make sure you educate yourself about this. Someone at work used to say, "It's your age. I get like that." They were either trying to be supportive or were avoiding the topic. I walked away shaking my head because the comment wasn't as comforting as she thought it would be. As someone with chemo brain, I have accepted it, but I had to realize that the people around me couldn't relate to chemo brain, so they used what they thought I could relate to.

Even after I finished chemo and radiation and returned to work, there were moments when things escaped me. A policy I had written, emails I had sent, or phone calls I had made were locked in my chemo brain.

I could never tell when I would face the loneliness of a past of which I had only fuzzy recollections.

I also experienced the loss of strength in my hands; just opening and closing them became an ordeal. I lost the endurance to brush my teeth, take a shower, go to work all day, shop, cook, clean, and care for myself and my family. A very thoughtful person at work gave me arnica cream for my hands. The littlest things can be the most thoughtful. Arnica helps with pain, and it's non-toxic.

At one point, I could not drive. I couldn't be trusted to stay on the right side of the road, drive in a straight line, and turn my head without feeling so out of balance that the trees along the side of the road looked like they were spinning. The biggest loss was independence. So I learned to be patient.

It took three years after surgery and treatment before I got to the point of being able to balance all the activities in my life that I had previously taken for granted.

When you finish chemo, the next hurdle is radiation. I saw the radiation oncologist first. She explained everything from what would be done to how, and reviewed the questions I had. She introduced me to the team, a nurse and three techs. These are very special people, highly skilled and professional with a dose of compassion for you. They loved my hats. I had become a hat maven because to me, wigs were ridiculous, and I couldn't manage with the fatigue brought on by dealing with them, so hats it was! They had a special place for my hat during each treatment.

Radiation was very difficult. It was the first time I had to physically expose my chest and be in the same room with my cancer, looking up at the ceiling to the rays that were ensuring the cancer cells would be removed, as well as other cells. The room was stark white and freezing cold. You are not permitted to move a muscle once they get you in position. They had music blaring. It was the only time I cried. I wasn't in pain, but I was cold, alone, and facing my cancer. The treatment lasted ten to fifteen minutes, and they radiated three areas. It was very powerful. When you are getting chemo there are other people and distractions. No distractions during radiation. It was therapeutic.

Mean Little Pill With A Pretty Name

So you get through the chemo and the radiation, and now it's on to this little pill you must take, an aromatase inhibitor. You take it if you have estrogen positive cells. The drug removes the estrogen that is produced in your organs so the cancer cells can't adhere to it. It is chemo-like, and that is a very simple explanation, because it is a complex pill. I took Femara. Don't be fooled by the tiny size of this medication with the pretty name. It packs a mean wallop.

I had never felt so bad in my life. Every bone in my body hurt. I wasn't sure if it was the pill or something else. When I woke up in the morning, my hands hurt. My feet hurt. I am now familiar with every joint in my feet because they all hurt at one point. When my back wasn't aching, it was racked by spasms that rippled through my body in wave after unceasing wave.

If I were seated, I would start squirming in my chair, which led to having to stand up, and the color would drain from my face. Try as I might to conceal what I was feeling by bullying myself and acting as if I was not having spasms, someone was always there saying, "Are you okay?"

You eventually get tough with yourself. I would have it out with myself. "You wimp, toughen up! Oh, you're exaggerating

— it's not that bad." After I stopped whipping myself, I took another path. I stopped feeling sorry for myself.

Nighttime was the worst. I hated when darkness came. I was so tired, but I knew what might be coming, so I tried to get to such a point of exhaustion that I would conk out quickly and sleep through the pain, but the leg spasms that jolted me awake and brought me to writhing and crying were my frequent nighttime companion.

Never have I experienced anything so bad — ten to fifteen minutes of sheer agonizing, unrelenting pain from my toes to my thighs. I squeezed Jimmy's hands until he begged for a break. I gripped the blankets as if I was falling off a cliff.

When it was over, I was afraid to move for fear of it returning, and sometimes on just a slight movement it would return.

During the day, I had spasms, but not just in my back. Sometimes my intestines cramped up, and the next thing I was in the bathroom for repeated visits. It got so bad that I was frequently dehydrated. This led to another round of speculation. Maybe I was magnesium depleted. Maybe my potassium was low. So I started taking vitamins and supplements.

What had I done to deserve this? Why was this happening? Everyone at home had a theory. You are working too many hours in a row. Maybe you are dehydrated. The list of suggestions went on and on.

The nightly spasms led Jimmy to do research. He was clearly upset watching me. So he found a remedy, and one night while I was in the middle of a spasm, he ran and got mustard and told me to inhale it, so I did, slow deep breaths, and it worked. OMG! Could this really be true?

While most people have flowers or books on their nightstand, I had a bottle of mustard.

One day I was at my neighbors' house visiting for a few hours. It was daytime, and I was sitting comfortably in a chair when I felt the spasm start, and I thought *Oh my God, what am I going to do?*

My neighbor clearly saw my distress. I tried to get up, but I couldn't stand, so she asked what she could do. I asked her for mustard. She went and got it while I explained why I needed it. From that point on, I traveled with mustard packets. After all, I was leaving for Florida the next day, and if I got a spasm on the plane, I needed a quick solution!

Life sure has changed. I began to use meditation tapes on my iPod at night. I would do anything just to sleep and relax a little. But the spasms never slowed down, or waxed or waned. So I had to mention it to my doctor. This was not only affecting my sleep; now it was carrying over into my daytime hours and encroaching on my life. I was feeling the effects of never being rested. Maybe I was a little cranky too.

It was the Femara causing the spasms, and something had to give. Did I want this drug to take over and rule who I was? I thought long and hard, and decided maybe I'd had enough of it. I was weary.

On my next visit to my oncologist, I brought the matter up. I realized this was not going to be easy. This was the man who had told me my medication plan could change based on the protocols known at the time. "I may keep you on it for life if it's going to keep the cancer from returning," he had told me. Somehow, I remembered hearing that.

I explained that I would like to come off the Femara. I explained that I had tried to cope with the side effects, tried to ignore them, thought I was crazy. I told him the whole story. He listened intently, nodded his head in acknowledgement, and said he had a suggestion. He thought I should take an antispasmodic, two milligrams at night. "You will sleep and not have spasms," he assured me, and then he added, "because we are not stopping the Femara, I can change it to another AI, but you need to be on it."

I thought about the fact that every decision I'd made regarding my breast cancer was to go for the best outcome, so how could I give up on Femara? It seemed reasonable to try the antispasmodic and see if it worked. And you know, it did. I still had spasms from time to time, but eventually they became less frequent, and that little white pill helped me sleep.

So I stayed on the Femara. I learned to cope with it. I didn't leave home without my antispasmodic, and I looked forward to taking it. Now that was a change — sounds like coping to me. I wish I had trusted myself more, and brought it up sooner — another lesson learned.

Fatigue

I had never really thought much about fatigue. In my years as a nurse, I never noticed how debilitating it could be for the patients I cared for, though I knew my role was to conserve their energy and provide frequent rest periods. I observed them to be weary and lacking energy, just as the definition of fatigue states, but I had no idea how different fatigue was from mere tiredness or even exhaustion. In the past, I had never really used the word in reference to how I felt. I may have said "I am so tired" or "I am exhausted," but I never referred to myself as fatigued. I didn't really relate to the word.

My cancer taught me many, many things. One of the most cherished lessons is that words have new meanings. I learned to understand what fatigue really means and how it works. When you look up the word in the dictionary, you find there are all kinds of fatigue, such as combat or battle fatigue — and when I read that, I thought *now we are getting closer to what it means when you have cancer fatigue*. So now, words have new meaning to me.

I had never really thought about the meaning of words. Maybe in the heat of the moment, I might have used a specific word to convey a particular message, but I had never really thought about the day-to-day meaning and impact of words. I love to communicate, and I value the process of communication. I try to be clear when speaking, and I always try to use the right words to convey my intended message, but this word *fatigue* was different because it encompassed the bone-deep feeling of having no energy whatsoever in my body.

Cancer fatigue is not tangible; it's insidious, and it really does sneak up on you and grab hold of you. It doesn't just take you by surprise — it takes you by force, literally and figuratively. I am not sure where I went in the midst of my fatigue, but I was gone in presence, gone in thought. It almost hurt, it was so real: you were there, and then you were not. Everyone else was there, so where did I go? Part of me felt robbed. I was no longer aware of what was going on around me. I was in the middle of a sentence or trying to get a thought out, and all of a sudden — I was gone, eyes closed, in my own world, but going nowhere.

It's almost like being in suspension somewhere. I remember people saying to me, "Go rest." They meant well, and I could hear them saying, "She needs the rest." Here's the next lesson: there is no resting with fatigue. Now that's an oxymoron. You lay down fatigued, and open your eyes fatigued. It's like a state of being. In the past, even when I was exhausted, I could push myself to keep going. When the kids were little and there was a communion party and so much preparation to be done, despite the fact that I felt so tired, I could push myself and know that I would make up for it later — but not with fatigue. You literally cannot push yourself, and that's a very foreign feeling if you've been strong and energetic your whole life.

I scolded myself to no avail. *What is so wrong with me that I can't even push myself? I am crumbling . . . how can I be so weak of mind and spirit?*

I eventually learned it's not that at all. Chemo takes your blood and shakes it up. Some cells are overtaken, and the oxygen-bearing cells cannot carry the oxygen like they normally do, and it makes you weary. The toxins created this fugue state, not me. They had taken over in a most powerful way. I couldn't fight it; after all, that would usurp more energy, so I learned to let it be, to give in, and I lived in a world of fatigue. Whenever I felt strong enough to be present, I would be, but I began to recognize fatigue for what is was, an all-encompassing beast, and eventually we got along together, and there was no more fighting it. I succumbed to fatigue.

Brushing my teeth, washing my face, and getting dressed had now become work, these mundane tasks that I always took for granted. Daily life changed. I could barely get that done, let alone make a morsel to eat or walk to the bathroom without help. My new normal became, *How am I going to get from one place to the next?* I actually calculated it: *If I do this, then I'll have to wait. Can I do something on my way to going somewhere else? Hmm . . . I might be able to do it.* I learned what conserving energy really meant.

Fatigue seems to have no beginning and no end. It took a long, long time for the fatigue to lift. When it's lifting is when you learn the different levels of fatigue. I would try to have a plan for the day, try and get to work, but once I was there, I needed to rest before I could do my job. Then I had to rest again before I could get myself home. I needed to rest again before I tried to eat dinner and prepare for the next day. Now my whole meaning of work changed. I never really thought of caring for myself as work. You never really think about these things until you have to. You just take it all for granted until it's gone.

So many times I tried to ignore the fatigue. The time I remember the most was at work. I would be keeping a steady pace and sailing along when all of a sudden, I would just bottom out. When this happened, it was frightening to me, but even more frightening was the look on the faces of my coworkers. There was no concealing it from them. In my pre-cancer days, some people might have noticed if I was tired, but that was the end of it. Now people looked at me with worried concern in their eyes, and I knew I was at the bottom, and try as I might to recover and move forward, I couldn't. So I learned patience. I had no choice. I had to succumb to the fatigue whether I wanted to or not, because it took over anyway.

I remember the day I decided to challenge fatigue. I looked it right in the eye and said, "I am tired of this bullshit. Today I am going out for a walk." It was close to zero degrees, there was snow on the ground, but I was tired of fatigue, so sick and tired of it controlling my life, and I was going to show fatigue not to reckon with me.

So, I put on my coat and was determined to walk around the block. I could do it. Off I went out into the biting cold. My cheeks hurt it was so cold. By the time I reached the corner, I realized I was walking like I'd had too much to drink.

In order to walk straight I had to concentrate on my steps and stay focused. That took nearly all of my energy. I turned back, determined to complete my task, and when I passed our firehouse, I decided I really needed to get inside because I was frozen. So I went into the post office.

There was nowhere to sit. I warmed up and headed out, changing my course. I would go to the bagel shop; it had tables and chairs. Got there and it was closed. Even colder now, I went into the flower/gift shop.

Our friend, Kathy, was happy to see me. I was happy to be warm, but, again, there was nowhere to sit. And to think I had to walk back home!

No cellphone either — I forgot to bring it (thank you, chemo). I couldn't call anyone to come and get me. So I warmed up, leaned against a few displays to rest my weary self, and then I headed out for home.

I got to the corner, and I was never so happy to see our neighbor Joe coming toward me.

I was in the road waffling side to side, and he took my arm, mentioned he saw me leave my house, and was a little worried. I can't imagine what I must have looked like when I left the house. I must've been quite a sight for him to come out after me on this freezing cold day!

I was so relieved. Now I knew I would make it home with his help. Arm-in-arm, we headed for our street. I was never so happy to be home, and I was so grateful for my kind neighbor. I got in, and my cheeks were so red and raw they looked like apples.

I have to say that was one of the stupidest things I did while suffering from chemo brain. I didn't fess up right away to my family about my escapade. It was my secret for now.

I learned a valuable lesson that day. You can't fight this disease on your own.

Eileen The Survivor

How can you move from fatigue to survivor? It's the natural course of events. As you crawl your way out of fatigue, you gradually remember who you are and why you feel this way, and you remind yourself that this is all part of moving toward good health.

But survivorship was work. Survivorship is fraught with pressure.

You are pressured to think you have come through this illness as a whole person and not the sum of your losses. You are even pressured into acceptance.

Acceptance came easier, however. I gave up thinking that everything that made me who I was before I got cancer would come back, so I accepted the new me. I was okay with it; after all, I am a survivor, aren't I?

There is that word again, survivor. Not always such a positive word.

I used to question how survivor and acceptance could be in the same sentence.

The day my doctor said, "Eileen, you are a survivor," he caught me off guard. The funny thing is, I had never really dwelled on the meaning of those words before, but now, when he said that, I thought, *Are you crazy? He must be crazy! A survivor doesn't feel the way I do. Doesn't he know I am not the person I used to be? I still feel like crap. How can he say that I am a survivor?*

I had not really thought of myself as a survivor, but now that I had, there were no bells, no fireworks, no feeling of joy or celebration. In fact, I couldn't even respond to his statement, something I regret to this day.

I felt pressure to say something, but words failed me. Instead of feeling elation at being deemed a survivor, I was dumbfounded by his pronouncement.

I didn't exhibit even a simple gesture of appreciation for what my doctor had done in anointing me a survivor.

So, a day or two later, I wrote my feelings down in a note to him. This was an unexpected lesson for me, one of the gifts you get from cancer that you only realize when you think about it later.

As a nurse, I always thought I was so lucky and privileged to become a part of a patient's life. After all, patients get very intimate with you in almost no time at all despite the fact that you are a complete and total stranger. This is something I love about my work and respect completely. But I never really considered how physicians feel about their work. I never thought they were as lucky as I was to bond so closely with patients. When I saw physicians making rounds in the hospital, it never seemed like they had the same impact on their patients that I had as a nurse.

My doctor guided me through this process. He always took my symptoms seriously. I will never forget him giving me that

look as I was leaving his office, the look that says, *I am sorry for what you are going through*. He squeezed my arm, and I felt his compassion in that gesture. It still haunts me that he was so in the moment and so concerned for the change he saw in me.

He acknowledged my loss; he saw the difference that cancer had made in my life. Even after all those years and all those cancer patients in between, he paid attention to me and to everything I was going through.

But he had eradicated the cancer. Those bastard cells were gone because of his knowledge and perseverance. Despite all the side effects, he kept pushing to get rid of those cells that were eating me alive, while I was only partially aware of what he was doing.

He cared enough to say, "Eileen, I know what this is doing to you, but we are going to push forward." And when he did have to stop the chemo for a while, he had a look of worry, which I can only now acknowledge.

At the time, I think I was just happy for the break and thought of it as a gift. I took that break. I was so grateful to have a moment or two from the punishing and grueling work of the chemo. What I didn't realize was that he bore the burden of putting off the chemo to give my body a chance to regroup.

He knew the risk involved; he calculated the risk and worried for me, and gave me a break from worrying, too.

I was so exhausted I never really was able to recognize his concern. I needed the break to survive. And I never acknowledged what he had done to get me to this point of being a survivor.

However, the day I gave him my note, he acknowledged the gift I gave him, and I was so grateful I had taken the time to do it. In my note, I expressed my appreciation for all he had done. In doing so, I gave myself a gift too.

Being appreciative of being a survivor was just one more thing I had to learn that I resisted learning because it is a reminder of what I went through and continue to go through. It is weighty, burdensome. I have to do it right, survive. You know me — suppose I don't do it right?

So here's the burden. What if I don't survive?

How long is a good survival time? Is that ever defined in medical terms or philosophical terms?

I don't want to fail at being a survivor. Wouldn't that be horrible? So you learn to accept the title, and I hope I can accept that when the time comes, it comes. I guess you can be a survivor more than once.

So much work to this survival business. Can you be tired of surviving?

But the true burden for me is that I don't like to be labeled.

I think that is really the problem for me. I did nothing grandiose to deserve this Survivor title. Heck, I barely was fully present. I think most survivors work at it; consciously, they have a plan and really work it. I wasn't like that.

You know who the survivors really are? All of those who helped me through it.

Those of you who did this for me, you know who you are. You worried through all of it.

After surgery, you helped care for me when I couldn't do it alone. You took me to my chemo treatments and my physical therapy three times a week.

You took me through snow and sleet. You stayed with me in the hospital, visited me in the emergency room to make sure everything was going okay, visited me when I was admitted. You flew in to stay with us and reassure me. You had patience with me when I was impatient with you. You made my bed, changed my sheets, stopped in to visit and chat, only to watch me sleep. You bought me a new bed and a new pillow so I could be comfortable now that I was unable to get out of bed for long periods. You took me to the hospital when I was so weak.

You offered words of encouragement, brought wine glasses for me and my friends so we could share a glass of wine over the phone. You sent food, and you made food for my family.

You reikiied me at home and from afar. You called and sent cards and flowers. You let me work at my own pace. You never forgot who I was, and that I could still contribute.

Best of all is that you helped my family cope.

You waited to hear the pronouncement, survivor!

You heard the bells and whistles even if I did not. You responded with a gentle sigh of relief.

I only went along for the ride because I had no other choice. You had lots of choices, but you chose to be there for my family and me.

I am in the game now to survive, but the real title goes to all of you who survived along this journey with me, and kept me inspired to survive with you.

I am so very grateful for the survivors in my life and for being able to share my gratitude with you.

Jimmy Reflects On Eileen's Diagnosis

The Fourth of July weekend in 2010 started for us on Friday, July 2, by driving our son Bryan to New York's JFK airport. Bryan was going to London as part of a study abroad program at Fordham University. He would be at the University of London for most of the summer and return shortly before he began his senior year.

Despite the holiday weekend, Eileen and I were able to go to and from the airport quite easily. The holiday traffic on the Long Island Expressway was not bad at all. We even made a side trip to get a few things for the weekend.

Like most of our July 4th holidays, this one was uneventful and ended nearly as soon as it began.

That year, the first day back at work provided the fireworks.

Tuesday, July 6, was not a bad day. By that I mean I was able to commute on the Long Island Rail Road quite easily as vacation season had begun in earnest and ridership was down. I was able to read my iPad and listen to the music on my iPhone with little or no interruption.

I had a peaceful day at work and arrived home at my usual time of 8:15 p.m. As soon as I entered the house, I felt the tension. Little did I know that my life was about to change and would never be the same again.

I have to say that when I get home from work, I'm usually low-key because I've had three hours to decompress on the train ride home. So, even if things are stressful at home before I arrive, I can handle it without exploding like Ralph Kramden in the 1950s TV show *The Honeymooners*.

This day was different.

I wasn't in the door five seconds when Eileen asked me to sit down because there was something she needed to tell me. This was an odd greeting, and I could sense there was something wrong with Eileen. I just didn't know how wrong.

The next thirty minutes are still a blur in my memory to this day. The only thing I remember is that she told me she had breast cancer, and the prognosis wasn't good.

Now, at this time I had been living with CLL for nearly ten years. That never scared me. I never felt that my world had imploded or turned upside down. Physically and emotionally, I felt the same way I had felt before the diagnosis. Even after ten years of dealing with it and two separate bouts of chemo, I felt in control and confident that all would be well.

The moment Eileen told me she had breast cancer, that all changed. I was no longer confident. I was no longer in control. I felt like I was dying.

It would be months later, long after her mastectomy and the early stages of her harsh chemotherapy, that Eileen would remind me of the difference between being a patient and a caregiver. She'd had ten long years of being my caregiver. Sure, I can say I felt strong and confident throughout my illness, but she knew better because she had suffered all the angst and concern that I was now experiencing as her soon-to-be caregiver.

I may offend some people, and I apologize in advance. One of the things that I learned while reading blogs and listservs is that CLL patients vary as to the severity of their symptoms and their experience with chemotherapy.

Many CLL patients suffer tremendously and do not respond to therapies, and eventually succumb to the disease. I am fortunate. I currently have an indolent form of CLL and, while I have required chemo and monoclonal therapy over the years, my disease is progressing very slowly. So, when I state that what Eileen experienced in her ordeal with breast cancer makes my bout with CLL seem little more than fighting a cold, I do not mean to minimize the beast that is CLL but merely to highlight my good fortune, so far, in dealing with the disease. I am also fully aware how quickly that can change.

I never had to exhibit the courage that Eileen was forced to display from the moment she learned of her diagnosis. As a nurse, she knew what she was in for. I had the luxury of ignorance to protect me during my first few weeks.

Eileen, on the other hand, knew she was gearing up for a life-threatening battle beginning with a radical bilateral mastectomy.

She would then have to deal with chemotherapy that would debilitate her and cause her to lose her hair. She dealt with that prospect by shaving her head before it had a chance to fall out. I never had to face any of that. I gained weight. That's about it. I gained weight.

To be fair to myself, I may never have had to endure what Eileen endured, but I had to watch. To be honest, I don't know how I was able to. Maybe my denial of my own condition extended to the coping behaviors I exhibited concerning hers. Maybe I just couldn't fathom what was happening. Maybe I just couldn't face the concept of losing her.

I don't know.

What I do know is that I had to be strong. I couldn't fall apart because Eileen wouldn't be able to put me back together, and what's worse, she might fall apart too. So we decided to laugh.

Well, first we cried. Then we planned to see her surgeon on the following Monday.

Now that I was in the loop, we had to discuss what to do next. Sean and Jeannine were both living and working in the Bronx, and I guess Eileen told them over the phone. We told the rest of our extended family the same way. Sean and Jeannine planned to come back out to East Quogue for the weekend. There was a festival on the North Fork in Cutchogue, and we were going to make a day of it.

Telling Bryan posed a difficult decision. Should we tell him over the phone while he was in England with no family nearby?

We couldn't delay telling him until he came home because Eileen would have had her surgery by then, and might even have started chemo.

Fortunately, technology provided a partial solution. We used Skype to video chat with him.

Bryan could see that his mom was in good spirits and exhibiting confidence, and we hoped this would help him absorb the shock without it overwhelming him. As we met with him via computer, with all of us chiming in, we hoped that he heard and saw that we had every reason to believe a successful treatment was possible.

Still, you worry.

As if we needed a reminder, cancer is not just an individual's disease. It affects everyone who loves you.

Come Monday

We had the appointment with Eileen's surgeon set for Monday morning, and the prospect of that was an albatross weighing me down.

Before anyone arrived at our house that Saturday, Eileen left me alone and decided to go to the farmers' market, just another typical summer Saturday. Well, I love Jimmy Buffet. I regularly listen to the *Margaritaville* radio program on XM radio, and on that particular day, moments after Eileen left to go shopping, the song "Come Monday" started playing.

I had to get up immediately and lock the door. I didn't want anyone coming in catching me crying. It was all I could do to stop long after the song ended. To this day, I cannot hear that song without welling up with tears.

When Eileen came home, I told her what had happened, and we had a tearful laugh at our situation.

A few minutes later, our good friends Vinnie and Maryann came in. We had a full house as the kids were there, of course, with the exception of Bryan, who was probably in Scotland sampling what that country is best known for.

We were all ready to go to the festival, but Vinnie wanted to pray with us before we left. Vinnie had been our parish priest back in the day at Blessed Sacrament in the Bronx. He is, in fact, featured in my first book *A Bronx Boy's Tale.*

We all gathered in our living room, and Vinnie began to pray. Fortunately, everyone had their eyes closed, so no one saw my heaving shoulders as I fought to keep from crying. Eileen saw it, of course, and came over to comfort me.

She was facing surgery and harsh chemotherapy, and she knew exactly how bad it was going to be, and she was comforting me!

Don't ever complain about nurses to me. They are superheroes.

You Know It When You Feel It

When you feel something is not right in your body, pay attention. Be present. Follow your gut feeling. Do your homework. But most of all, be brave and have faith.

When I was diagnosed with breast cancer in 2010, Jimmy was already ten years into his relationship with Dr. Avvento and Eastern Long Island Hematology and Oncology. Because of this, Jimmy automatically assumed I would choose his team to treat my illness.

This is where my belief system kicked in. If you need to rely on others, choose wisely and make sure they are people you trust. Take your time to know what you want. Spend time getting to know yourself. Be honest with yourself and your feelings. Your belief system will guide every decision you make. You must trust yourself so there will be no doubts. The message here is YOU make the decisions, not your doctor. It's a weighty decision — you get to do this once. Get it right.

I was now in the healthcare system, not as a provider, but as a patient.

I went for my mammogram feeling certain I was going to encounter a problem. I just didn't think it would happen so quickly. It was abrupt, actually, like a conversation with someone who bites you when they speak.

The radiology department at Southampton Hospital where I worked did everything to make a mammogram as comfortable as possible. The radiology staff was professional and sensitive to my need for privacy. That was so important to me as I prepared for the procedure.

Pick your place of diagnosis very carefully. Do your homework. Research the equipment in use, and learn about the staff and physician.

I made it through the initial procedure but needed more tests. It was during the breast sonogram that there was certainty regarding my diagnosis.

Chet and I had worked together at another hospital, and I knew that he was always very gentle and kind. I really appreciated that about him. Funny thing — I wasn't suspicious when he said he was writing notes, and that I should stay where I was.

In came the next member of the team, the radiologist. He was clear and concise. He showed me the films and outlined the problem.

I appreciated that because from that moment, I knew that I had decisions to make.

His last words were, "Leave no stone unturned, Eileen." And then, he said the most incredible thing. "Here is my cell phone number. I will be in the mountains on vacation, but if your children or husband want to talk to me, have them call this number."

This was more than I could ever have expected. This is a man who cares, who knows what you need so you don't even have to ask for it.

People can and do the unexpected at a most unexpected time. Pay attention to those moments; they are the gift of cancer.

The radiologist has an important job. He (or she) is the first one who gets to see your cancer cells, and in my experience, there was no delay on his part.

I chose a breast center for diagnosis and treatment because there was a team of practitioners that I trusted. There was a breast surgeon, a radiologist, nurses, techs, and secretaries, all part of the coordination of care. For me, this was a very positive experience.

Unfortunately, when I was having the mammogram, my soon-to-be breast surgeon was away, hence the radiologist gave me the proposed diagnosis. (Try not to have your diagnosis made on the Friday of the Fourth of July weekend!)

When I met with the breast surgeon, she provided an unrushed atmosphere. I urge you to go to your appointment with questions, not answers. Be open to discussions of why and why not. The better informed you are, the better your decisions about taking whatever steps come next.

Get a second opinion, but know your facts before you go to that appointment. If you are not a listener, now is when you must learn to listen.

With that in mind, I went in to New York City for my second opinion. I met with a nurse practitioner who took a very detailed history, and then the consultant physician came in and got right to the exam. She reviewed my treatment plan as outlined by my surgeon, and she wasn't in agreement. She told me why.

I had opted for a bilateral mastectomy, and she advised chemo first. Her reasoning: shrink the tumor and then do surgery.

I explained I wanted to proceed this way because I had areas of concern on my right side. After I said this, she indicated that she had not viewed my films. Her radiologist had.

She asked for the films, but her staff had a hard time locating them. I left knowing I would definitely not be using their services.

I called my breast surgeon on the way home. I was a bit unnerved and uncertain as to whether my decision might be flawed. My surgeon took the call, and the conversation was very reassuring.

Having a belief system is what you will fall back on every single time, especially when making decisions. You have to know where you want to go on this journey. Will you have surgery? Will you undergo chemotherapy and radiation? You can't make it up as you go. My breast surgeon knew that I was leaning toward a double mastectomy, and she knew why. That was key. Now it was time to see the oncologist.

I called in a favor from a friend and got in to see my soon-to-be oncologist. I had known Dr. Avvento for quite a few years and never thought I would be one of his patients.

He saw me at the end of the day. What I noticed right away was that he listened. Actually, he said very little. Once the final tests were in, I would be going back for decision-making. When that day came, I had my daughter come with me, and she took notes.

He never batted an eye that she was recording his advice. I can't tell you how many times I had to refer to those notes. It was very helpful. If you can have someone accompany you when you are getting treated, it is a good idea. Only bring someone you trust who is also a good listener. Choose wisely.

He laid out the options, and I was shocked. I could decide? Are you kidding me? How do you do this when you are so vulnerable? The next lesson you learn is that you will make the decision.

This is a very personal thing. It's your body. Take your time, but make the decision and know why you're making it.

I wanted the best outcome. At every step of the way, I had to ask: What will give me the best outcome? What will the surgery or treatment do to me physically and emotionally?

I told very few people about my diagnosis until I made my decision. I had to be comfortable with my decision, and I needed to know why I made it and whether it made sense to do it. People try to be helpful, but in reality, some people are very unhelpful, another thing you have to deal with.

Dr. Avvento sent me to get a second opinion regarding the treatment after surgery.

When you get a second opinion, be sure to bring your primary doctor's recommended plan with you. My consulting oncologist had my films as well as the treatment plan for chemo and radiology.

He agreed with everything Dr. Avvento recommended. He said he would follow the same plan. That was very reassuring.

He was open, honest, and actually very helpful. He gave me great advice.

Then there's chemo.

Dr. Avvento laid out the plan, and he had me meet his team. Before you can receive any treatment, you will meet the team who will be there for you during the extent of your treatment.

I have already described how kind he was to me when I was struggling with the treatment. He gave me a break when I really needed it, but he continued to worry about letting me have that break.

Radiation was harder on me emotionally than chemo was. This was when the team was so crucial to my recovery. Radiation therapy requires such precision and the proper alignment of the body and the ray to ensure that the radiation is directed at the cancer cells. I never felt as if I was just the next patient. I WAS the patient. They were so respectful of me.

Friendship Defined

Jimmy

It may seem counterintuitive that something good can come out of a cancer diagnosis.

Certainly, no one wants to get cancer regardless of any positive experiences the patient and family may enjoy. However, one of the things I encountered when I first got that phone call was that my priorities began to realign themselves within seconds.

All the things that were important the day before were flipping and flopping like pachinko balls on steroids.

All the stress associated with work not only got pushed to a back burner — it wasn't even allowed to stay in the kitchen. I couldn't care less if our automated financial aid system blew up.

It was exhilarating.

I was free from the banal and mundane. When you are staring at your own mortality, the prospect of your boss getting on your case no longer concerns you. But the freedom from work-related angst was far from the most significant emotion I experienced.

We all know about fair-weather friends, but we rarely talk about our foul-weather friends.

Here are some of ours.

If you are blessed to have longtime friends, I'm sure you know the feeling that no matter how long it has been since you've seen each other, the moment you hear each other's voice, whether in person or on the phone, you pick up right where you left off the last time you spoke.

It could be years since you last spoke, but you are able to reconnect as you did back in the day. Let me tell you about my friends who have been there for me through foul weather and fair, through good times and bad.

Mike, PJ, Freddy, Trent, and Lou have been in my life for over fifty years. Sometimes there have been huge gaps of time between our get-togethers. Mike and PJ worked in New York City where I worked, and getting together for a beer after work was something we tried to do one or two times a year.

Freddy was up in Rockland County and was not able to attend as many of these sessions as he would have liked. Trent and Lou were out of state and far away from New York. Nevertheless, in the last few years, we've all gotten together for a lost weekend at PJ's house out in Hampton Bays, New York.

When I was diagnosed, Mike and PJ had to deal with my news. It's funny how we are sometimes. Here I was the one with the leukemia, and I was worried about how they would take the news. Similar to the way I told my family, I downplayed the serious nature of my disease and said it was not only treatable, but I would probably live a normal life and die from something else.

Again, similar to my family, they didn't buy my story, and I could see the worry and concern in their eyes.

But one thing I have learned is that people take your lead and treat you the way they think you feel. I was my old gregarious self, still doing the things I had always done. We met for drinks after work, a couple of beers at the beach on a Saturday afternoon, and a countless number of Yankee and Jets games.

I didn't look any worse for wear, and I think that made it easier for all of us to accept that, while I had cancer, I seemed to be doing pretty well, and that was reassuring.

When I was going through chemo, it was more of the same in terms of how I dealt with CLL and what I allowed others to see. One thing I have to confess is that, while I think I did present a good front, I have absolutely no way of knowing how effective I was in making everyone think I was okay. I am not even sure I convinced myself of that, but I never questioned it. I believed I was okay, and I really think I was.

Chemo caused me to gain twenty-five pounds both times I was in treatment. The first course was in 2000, and I went from 225 pounds to 250. Then, in 2007, I went up to 275 pounds. I always blamed the chemo for this weight gain, but I would also add that it might have been the Twinkies. (I haven't had a Twinkie in forty years, but I just had to make a joke.)

Joking was my thing, and I thought that would help others deal with my CLL. I fully accept that it may only have allowed me to deal with it.

Whether I was fooling my friends or myself or not, phone calls were made and emails were sent just to make sure I was doing okay. Distance is no barrier in the digital communication age, and that was a blessing.

The Bronx Boys may have been separated geographically, but data bytes knew no barrier of time or distance, and we might as well have been on Hoch's Corner on Leland Avenue when it came to keeping in touch.

Some friends were more compulsive when it came to keeping in touch and checking in. Our friends Pat and Paul would not accept phone call or email assurances. Pat, in particular, had to see for herself. You also could not deliver a week's supply of dinners via electronic means. So, every Sunday of the week I would be undergoing chemo, Paul was compelled to drive from River Edge, New Jersey, out to East Quogue, a distance of more than one hundred miles each way, just to placate his wife Pat so that she could rest easily knowing that I would have enough to eat. This, perhaps, might be the real reason for my propitious weight gain.

The thing you have to understand is that Paul traveled all week to and from various locations within the country and sometimes throughout the world. He actually had more frequent flyer miles than Neil Armstrong. I am sure that after a long week of work and travel, Paul would have much rather been watching his New York Giants in the comfort of his living room. But you would never know that if you saw him with Pat at our house on these Sunday visits.

We laughed and joked as always, and while I was grateful for the food that was delivered, it was the love of the two people who brought the food that sustained me during that time.

New friends also were important to me. My staff at the schools where I worked during treatment always had my back. Then, when I went to Downstate, supervisors and colleagues, all true friends, supported me through my own battle and Eileen's as well.

Eileen

So many people helped us through my battle with breast cancer. I have been blessed with a terrific family and loving and loyal friends. It's important to acknowledge those feelings and recognize the value in them. This will sustain you.

Being a nurse, it is no surprise that most of my closest friends are nurses. From the girls I went to nursing school with to the colleagues who became lifelong friends, I truly have some fantastic women and men in my life.

Jimmy confided in me early on in my treatment that he felt left out. In trying to protect him, I did leave him out of some of the trips and treatments. The house was always filled with nurses, and he had little to do for me. I would change that if I could go back in time and do things differently, but I think my illness gave him coping skills he didn't have initially.

My brother Kevin and Eileen (my sister-in-law) often popped in to see how I was progressing. My brother Jimmy and Dorothy lived in the neighborhood and frequently popped in to offer food as well as strength through words of encouragement. My sister-in-law Maureen drove from Westchester to my house for a day of cooking while I pretty much slept on the couch. It was so thoughtful of her to do that. Karen DeSimone and Connie Andersen were with me when I got home from my surgery. In fact, that was their vacation week, and they spent it with us so that they could look after me. They had planned to spend a week with us anyway, but that was to go to the beach as we did every year. This year, they nursed me back from surgery and kept Jimmy's spirits up.

Pat Darcey — who I only call my boss because she is my boss, but in reality she is one of my dearest friends — got the hospital to put me in a private room, and she had it stocked with food and drinks for my family and friends who spent long hours at my bedside.

So many people were good to us, and we are so appreciative of the kindness of others.

Once the surgery was complete and I was on the mend, but before chemo treatments started, Pat put me on projects to keep me working and getting paid. I learned much later that she was suffering in silence, worrying about me and not wanting to let it appear to anyone that she was worried.

Then there was Pat Lowenwirth. Not only was she with me for every treatment, but she also came loaded down with a goody bag of dinners and treats to ensure that no one starved while I was not able to cook.

Traveling one hundred miles each way to be with me did not dampen her smile or inhibit her laughter. She made me feel better just being there.

It was truly wonderful to behold. So many kind and loving people went out of their way to tell me how much I was loved. Not that I took Jimmy for granted, but I was used to his love. He's loved me since I was seventeen.

People say that the only things you can depend on are death and taxes. Well, Jimmy's love for me can be tacked on to that list.

But being given the opportunity to see the love people had for me acted out in front of my eyes was the greatest blessing you could possibly imagine. I would need this love to get through the next few months, as they would not be pretty at all.

So I share my appreciation with all of you, my co-survivors, because you carried me through my illness and remain in my life today.

There Are No Coincidences

Eileen

Life takes you on a path. Where you are going, you have no idea. Who will accompany you has been decided. How you get there is part of the plan.

But what you learn along the way is up to you.

I believe that God is the author of the plan, and we can deny the plan, we can choose to go off course from the plan, but no matter what, that's part of the plan too.

This chapter is going to be very detailed because it is a significant part of how I became who I am and how my life's journey was all part of the Creator's plan.

My story is going to start from a point many years ago.

Growing up I always felt like all I wanted to do with my life was to be good, to help people, to make peace, and to simply be an authentic person.

I really felt there was a purpose to my life. Even as a young girl, when I really didn't know what the purpose was going to be, I knew it would be special.

Maybe it was because I was the youngest in my family, or maybe because I felt so loved, especially in my early years.

I was born when my mother was 45 and my father was 55. When I was a year old, my father died of cancer and renal failure. Of course, I didn't know what he died of, and for years, no one talked about it. I just assumed he had a heart attack, so when my friends asked me, that is what I said.

Nevertheless, despite this tremendous loss, I felt loved and cared for by my extended family and the many friends who supported my family.

I later learned that my mother took care of him during his illness, and my father died at home. My brother Patrick and my sister Mary, with the help of dear friends of the family, took care of her and the rest of my family, including me.

This was long before hospice or palliative care services were available. Even so, my mother wanted my father home, and that was it, no further discussion.

Even though I never got to know my father, I do remember feeling loved from a very early age because so many people helped to make up for his absence.

Empathy for others is a bond that lasts a lifetime. It kept us connected as families for years. They offered us the gift of love, kindness, and fun.

There were trips to Lake Sebago in upstate New York where we played softball and went swimming. Other times, people just filled in when my mother was working two jobs. Whatever needed to be done was done.

That is not to say that life didn't present its challenges for me. Even with all of that support, I never had much confidence in myself. I never considered myself smart, and I accepted that I wasn't.

Our neighbor and family friend Uncle Charlie used to tutor me in math. Oh, how I hated math. I never thought I could achieve greatness, so I never pushed myself, and did just enough to get by. Besides, I thought I really didn't need algebra to survive.

This became the metaphor of my teen years.

What I later grew to appreciate over the years was that just getting by is what you want to avoid. Work through the challenge. I also learned that you needed algebra too!

Because my mother worked two jobs, we were a busy family, and while it was important to go to school and do well, we were never really pushed to excel. If she were here now, she might not agree with that, but it's my interpretation (or excuse) for how I proceeded in school. She did make sure I took piano lessons, and later in life she told me she always wanted to be a baby nurse.

My mother believed that to do the best I could was what mattered. To me, school grades just didn't seem so important.

My mother left the house at ten in the morning and returned around midnight. Mary, my sister, went to high school at night so she could work during the day. She did the shopping and the cooking. She helped with homework and kept peace among the three of us. She gave her life to our family in ways no one can even imagine.

I try to remember that now. She took us to the movies, bought our clothes for school, and even made sure we covered our books for that first week of school. Mary was a superstar in that role.

Patrick, my older brother, was in college when I was in grammar school. When he finished college, he went to law school. He was the serious student of the family; the rest of us, not so much, until later.

He and Mary were about sixteen years older than me. I really don't remember much about Patrick from my early years. I remembered what the family pictures showed me.

I know he worked extra when I was small. And when he went college, he had different hours than I, so I don't remember too much of the early years.

I remember his friends and how they always met at our house before going off for a night of fun. Then he met Maureen, and they fell in love and were married on August 8, 1968.

I think that was the year I found out about his illness. My memory is that I was clowning around with him and hit him a little too hard on the leg.

Later that night Mary told me that Patrick had an illness. It was called Hodgkin's disease.

It never came up again for another four years. You'll see a connection soon.

When I was in high school, I hurt my knee. My brother Jimmy worked for the NFL and made a recommendation to see the New York Giants doctor who worked at St. Vincent's Hospital in Greenwich Village, New York City.

I had to have surgery, and while I was a patient at St. Vincent's, I fell in love with nursing — head over heels in love.

The nurses taught me everything. Who even thought that the knee could be so glamorous, but I was fascinated to learn and understand why they were going to fix my knee, how they were going to do it, and what the rehabilitation plan would be. That was so intriguing to me.

The nurses were great; they explained everything every time they tended to me. I felt so safe.

That was when the light bulb went off for me: *I am going to be a nurse, and I am going to be a St. Vincent's Hospital nurse!*

So where's the coincidence?

My brother Patrick went to a doctor at SVH long before I had the surgery and before I knew anything about his illness.

I went to nursing school with my best friend from high school, Pat Adams then, Lowenwirth now.

Nursing school was the best of times and the worst of times. So much studying to do, so much partying to do, all of it in Greenwich Village, an exciting place to be in New York City.

There were pre-conference preparations, post-conference preparations, and learning how to do things, and why you had to do them.

We had a beau parlor and a housemother. "Fetchie" kept a keen eye on us and the beau parlor, and Vincent the elevator man watched us like hawks while reciting, "Step lively!" when we got on the elevator. He was a jolly man, friendly, kind, and very obliging. I don't think I ever saw him crabby; he seemed so proud of his work.

My SVH experience filled my life, and Greenwich Village was my playground. I was so lucky to have such a great experience, and it shaped my life in ways unexpected.

So I mentioned that Patrick went to a doctor at SVH. Who was this man? I had to find out.

One day I took myself over to the research lab and we got acquainted. No HIPPA back then; patient privacy hadn't been invented yet. You could show up at a doctor's office and talk about a family member, which is what I did.

It was years later that I really understood that Dr. R was a research doctor. I always met him in his lab, a true scientific laboratory. I had no idea that he was doing research in the hospital. I worked there and never really understood that. Now I really get it. I would pop in every so often and just say, "How's it going?"

But first a little history.

Back when Patrick was in high school, he went home after playing football one day when my mother noticed a lump on his neck and assumed it was a football injury.

She was wise enough not to take it lightly and sent him to the doctor, who told Patrick it was either an infection or Hodgkin's disease.

They treated him for an infection, and it had no effect on the lump. The doctor was very concerned and sent him to see Dr. C who did a biopsy and confirmed the diagnosis. This happened a short while after my father died.

This is when Patrick began his fifteen-year relationship with Dr. R. Dr. R was a father figure to Patrick and supported him during his illness.

I get lost in thought sometimes and wonder how Patrick coped with all of this. His father died from cancer and now he had cancer. How could my mother cope with this?

Was there a relationship between my father's cancer and Patrick's?

You can imagine the impact that Jimmy's diagnosis had on me, and how my own diagnosis affected me. My life was connected by cancer.

I never got to ask Patrick how he coped. All too soon, our conversations took a more serious turn.

Time was running out.

Forty years ago, the only treatment for Hodgkin's disease was radiation. When Patrick was sick or undergoing treatment, he never spoke about what he was going through.

I really don't know what he thought all those years. I would love to know how he felt. I wish I could have heard it from his perspective. I got to know him and Maureen a little better at a time when it was obvious that Patrick was not feeling well.

I had graduated from St. Vincent's in 1975 and was working at SVH. The following year, Jimmy and I were married.

Things were going well when I noticed Patrick was losing weight. He was pale, shaky, and not himself. I noticed Maureen seemed strained, but she never said anything.

I was very concerned.

Patrick liked to paint and listen to classical music; sometimes I think he was a true renaissance man.

He did those things to express himself, but perhaps also to relax and distract himself from what was troubling him.

We shared a session together — painting that is. I liked to paint and considered myself capable, but I never really developed my technique.

I always enjoyed a particular day at Patrick and Maureen's home in Montrose, New York, when we had the easels and paints out, and Patrick was teaching me about burnt umber and all the available color choices.

It was a special day.

On another occasion, Patrick shared that he was getting discouraged. He was tired, yet he couldn't sleep. He didn't have the strength to shovel snow, nor could he do the simple things he had always done.

I could see he was upset, and maybe it was my imagination, but I thought Maureen was upset too, but she did not speak about it.

So I went to see Dr. R and asked what was going on with Patrick. I shared what Patrick had shared. Dr. R talked to me about how important nutrition was and how Patrick had to eat the right foods, and that he should get a juicer and begin juicing carrots and cabbage and anything green.

I left feeling flabbergasted that vitamins and vegetables were now going to be Patrick's frontline treatment. How could this help him?

Shortly thereafter, I received a call from Maureen. She said Pat had been to Dr. R, and Pat told him he was feeling down, had bad night sweats, wasn't sleeping, had no energy, and so on.

Dr. R prescribed a sleeping pill.

Maureen went to fill the prescription, and the pharmacist told her she could get this prescription filled or simply go over to aisle 8 and buy a bottle Tylenol.

Maureen didn't know what to do. I was as shocked as she was when she told me, but I got angry.

I went to see Dr. R and, boy, did he get a piece of my mind.

I was livid and asked him why he couldn't tell Patrick the truth. Furthermore, if he was so concerned about his health, why did he make Patrick's wife have to go through that?

I may have said other things, but I know that was the day I decided that we needed another plan here.

It took a while, but fortunately, Patrick's best friend Joe was of the same mind and had spoken to Patrick. So I made a suggestion that Patrick go for another opinion from Dr. G. at SVH to see what he could offer.

Eventually Patrick did, and he ended his relationship with Dr. R. We never really got into how that went. I know it must have been hard for Patrick to do that after so many years, very hard. But he wanted a better life. He owed that to his wife and children, and to himself.

Dr. G was Patrick's age, early thirties, and that made all the difference. He was a young, new oncologist full of energy, optimism, and skill. Patrick hit it off with him as well as the nurses. Patrick and I met up with each other quite often, but I wish I had asked him more questions about his illness and treatments.

When he had a doctor's appointment with Dr. G, we would meet for coffee, lunch, or just a quick chat. I worked across the street from the Maritime building on Seventh Avenue where Patrick had his treatments.

At this point in his illness, chemotherapy was an option. He seemed healthy, and was managing his treatments. I remember him talking about losing his hair and that they were putting a rubber band/tourniquet around his head to prevent hair loss. Dr. G would try anything new; he was always keeping up with the latest research.

Patrick was working, playing with the kids, planning trips, and enjoying life. It was good to see him back in the game. I know it could not have been as easy as I recall, but mostly he seemed happy again.

A few years later when the holidays were rolling around, we were going to have a bake-off, and fruitcake was on the menu. I think his came out better than mine.

I noticed that he didn't look well. He had really started to lose weight, and he looked pale and tired.

Shortly after Christmas, Patrick had an incident on his way to work. He was admitted to St. Vincent's.

Patrick was not always a great patient after a chemo regimen.

Patrick was a smoker too.

He was in the hospital a few days, and I was already getting worried. He wasn't progressing. I decided one night that I was going to stay with him.

A cardiologist told us that Patrick had endured some damage to his heart from the Adriamycin, and he had pleural effusions that were worsening, which necessitated a lung tap to remove the fluid.

I was definitely staying with him.

I brought up the subject of staying over, but Pat had another plan. After Maureen helped him to the bathroom and back again, Patrick told me that I was to go home with Maureen and pick up their kids, who were being cared for by their good friends Irene and Austin.

Patrick would arrange for a private duty nurse. I was not happy, but I knew he wanted someone with Maureen, so I did what he needed me to do.

Before we left, the lung tap was done, and they took out three liters of fluid.

We stayed a while and finally left at around 9:00 p.m. and headed to Montrose. Austin met us when we got off the train, and we went with him to get the kids from his house. As soon as we got to Maureen and Pat's house, the phone was already ringing.

I was settling the kids in their beds when I heard Maureen say, "You need to talk to his sister now."

I found out that he had coded, he was in intensive care on a respirator, and he had a chest tube. His lung collapsed after all the fluid was removed. He was critical but stable, but we needed to go back. We called Austin and Irene. We dropped off the kids with Irene, and Austin drove us back to the hospital.

So began Patrick's four and a half month ordeal in the ICU. That was the longest time in my family's life. When I think back, it was truly the best of times as much as it was the worst of times.

Those first few days in ICU must have been torturous for Patrick. In the beginning, he would attempt to get out of bed and had to be restrained. Every time he tried to get out of bed, he extubated the respirator (removed the tube), but then he could not breathe, so they had to re-intubate him.

He didn't know what he was doing; he would fall asleep, wake up, and take that thing that was in his mouth out.

Imagine seeing your thirty-six-year-old loved one tied up in restraints. I was scared but never let on. My concern was whether his breathing tube had been out too long. Was his brain receiving the necessary oxygen to survive?

How could this have happened? How did it all change in an instant? One week you are baking fruitcakes and the next you are fighting for your life.

Then it got worse.

Patrick had infections. Every Monday it was something different. He had two chest tubes, a feeding tube, a tracheotomy, IVs, and what seemed like a hundred transfusions. He was in isolation then out.

This is when I really began to use my nursing skills and when I learned the power of touch.

Human contact, touching, is crucial to living and preserving life. My hands were comforting. My technique was flawless. I could do what Patrick needed and do it with love and compassion. I was not a critical care nurse, but I knew he needed the critical care I could give: compassion, love, and touch.

I knew how to manage his lines, tubes, and vent. I got him bathed and changed his sheets, even while he was still in the bed.

I began to get him out of bed and into a recliner, which made all the difference because he was in ICU for four and a half months and never got a bedsore.

We got rid of his Foley and learned how to plug his tracheotomy so he could speak to us.

He was nutritionally compromised. At times, he had diarrhea. Nevertheless, when I left him at night he was snug as a bug, so comfortable, so clean. He felt good and I felt even better.

During some of those one-on-one sessions that I shared with Patrick, I talked and he wrote. He was very expressive in his writing, so clear. He amazed me.

In the early days, he was confused. I was so heartbroken, and then I worried that there was brain damage, but he rebounded and remained very clear.

We celebrated each holiday. Maureen and the kids would paint and draw, and his room was wallpapered with their art. We had St. Patrick's Day festivities and Easter too!

One day we arranged for the kids to visit him. Grandma came down with Maureen and the kids. Dr. G stopped to talk to the kids while they were with my mother. He told them, "I am going to make your daddy well." My mother was so upset by that. I know he believed what he said with all his heart. My mother was ahead of her time, I think, because she was very upset. I could see in her face what she was thinking: *Suppose he doesn't get well, and you promised those kids you were going to make him well?* My mother shared that with us later, but said nothing to the doctor at the time.

Megan crawled into the bed when she saw him. Kathleen just looked from the bottom of the bed. She was older and knew what fear was.

That visit by Patrick's kids was a hard day for us all, but it was also an exciting day because everyone was together again.

For Easter, we colored Easter eggs together, a keepsake his daughters have to this day.

I read up on how to preserve them. In those days crafting was my hobby, so I blew out the egg through a tiny pinhole, and after we colored them, we were able to save them.

At one point Patrick started to rebound, and there was even talk about his getting well enough to go home. I remember him talking to me about moving out to the Hamptons when he got out. He and Maureen had a summerhouse in Hampton Bays, and his plan was to sell that house to Jimmy and me, and he and Maureen would buy a bigger house.

During Patrick's entire hospital stay, we ran a shuttle from the Bronx to SVH in Manhattan and back again. Jimmy was the principal cabbie, but sometimes Peter was the driver or one of my brothers.

At one point, Dr. G was off, and another oncologist was covering his patients. He told us Patrick would not make it through the weekend.

Maureen was crushed by the news, but she had the good sense to tell this doctor that he needed to tell Patrick. "He has children, you know," she added.

The doctor was not in favor of this, but I remember Maureen persisted in fighting for Patrick's right to know. Maureen went in with the doctor, and they told Patrick together. I sat on a stretcher in the hallway waiting and wondering. How could all this be happening?

It was so surreal. Maureen came out and told me Patrick wanted to see me. I took a deep breath before going in. He told me not to worry. Nothing was going to happen this weekend. Dr. G would be back and he would know what to do. He would figure it out; he always did. I nodded and thought, *I have to do this for him*. Back in the hall, I felt bad for him because I did not share his belief. I knew he could leave us at any time.

When Dr. G returned, he saw me visiting Patrick and asked me to come to the desk. He got Patrick's chart, opened it, and said, "I don't know what to do."

He reviewed labs, X-rays, and meds, and was puzzled by Patrick's condition. I remembered what Patrick had said, and he was right: Patrick had made it through the weekend a few weeks ago! And of course Dr. G would know what to do.

I walked away feeling totally confident. I was so used to Dr. G figuring out what to do that I had no concern. I realized later the other oncologist was trying to tell me he really didn't know what else to do. I guess it was too hard to say that clearly, or maybe he was clear, but I just wasn't ready to hear it.

All through this ordeal there were so many times when I thought he wouldn't make it, but he did.

Eventually we got the message, and we all took turns staying overnight with him. We also began to plan the funeral. We all went to the cemetery to pick out the plot and meet with the undertaker to plan Patrick's final journey.

I remember the night before he died. My brother Kevin stayed with him, and I relieved Kevin.

That morning I knew Patrick was actively dying. The nurses were professional; the room was somber. I sat beside Patrick and talked to him, but I felt him pushing me out — that's the only way I can describe it. I had been saying the things you tell someone when you will never see them again.

I left the room and called home to let them know they should head down to the hospital if they wanted to be there. I returned to the room, and a little while later, I did not know why, but I wanted to get a drink. I again felt him pushing me out.

I told him I loved him and would be back in a few minutes. I looked at him before I left. He was thin, very still, not opening his eyes when he had always been so actively involved.

This was different.

He did not appear in pain. I left the room begrudgingly, but I did what he was willing me to do.

I came back and Mrs. L, the receptionist in ICU, said to wait a minute. I knew.

Now the doctor came, they called Father J., and they surrounded me. I just sat there — no tears, disbelief — then guilt.

I was supposed to be there when it happened, and that is when I realized he didn't want me there. I asked Father J. why I wasn't crying; this made no sense. How would I tell my family he was alone when he died?

He said, "Don't tell them. Why do they need to know?" So I didn't for many years, and then one day I let them in on the secret.

Now it was time to make a call, the final call from the ICU nurses' station. I called home and let them know. It was a long time before the tears came.

So here are the connections.

As a nurse, my work was to heal, help, and comfort others. I did most of that with my hands, with touch. I learned you had to touch to connect with a patient. The connection was just as important as the medications I administered.

I made a point of touching my patient's shoulder, maybe their hand or knee. I used my hands to bathe and provide comfort to the patient, comfort that the family could see.

I used my eyes to connect; you can learn a lot about a person by looking right into their eyes. You can see pain and suffering, especially when they are verbalizing that everything is okay.

Now I looked at my hands differently; I used them differently at home, and at work.

Things for me changed.

All My Life's A Circle

Thirty-one years after my brother Patrick died, I was diagnosed with cancer.

I was expecting it to arrive some day given my family history, but nonetheless, I was surprised.

And now, suddenly my life would be surgery, chemo, and radiation.

The surgery left me with lymphedema. I had so many changes to deal with, so many losses. Femara, the drug I had to take for five years, made every bone hurt, every step hurt. My body was wracked with aches and pains and cramps. My fingers hurt so severely that I couldn't bend my fingers. To this day, I have very little strength in my hands. I didn't realize how upset I was about my loss of dexterity until I fell and hurt my hand with the lymphedema.

I was almost panic-stricken to think that my hand might be broken. How would it heal?

That's when I made the connection to Patrick, and what my hands have meant to me all my life. All those years I took them for granted.

The entire experience with Patrick prepared me for the rest of my life.

It helped me when Jimmy was diagnosed, when my sister Mary was diagnosed with breast cancer a short time after Jimmy's diagnosis, and with my own diagnosis and treatment for breast cancer.

I had to take Adriamycin, just like Patrick, and I also had heart issues while taking it. One of the luckiest things for me was that the hospital I worked in had a wellness center, and this is where I learned about another connection, juicing and eating natural foods.

Patrick had that experience with his first doctor. Dr. R.'s research for Hodgkin's was all about the importance of nutrition, leafy green vegetables, and juicing, all the way back in the '70s when most doctors gave no thought to the impact of nutrition on disease. And now I was juicing, eating more natural foods, fewer processed foods. Another connection.

My brother's illness helped me to cope with my own, another example that there are no coincidences in life.

Imagine if I'd never had that experience. I would not understand the depth of comfort and healing in sharing, leaning on others, and being leaned on when they need you, the importance of touch, and how experiences such as these make the bonds of love stronger.

These experiences connected us and will always keep us connected. We learned to accept the good with the bad, and we continued to grow regardless.

We learned that you could survive even in the face of such insurmountable loss. These life lessons aren't taught at school. Reality was our teacher, and we were open to the lesson.

So here's the thing:

If you are not open, you cannot learn.

If you cannot learn, you miss the lessons in life.

If you miss these lessons, you can't help others.

The connections fail or are never made.

Of course, I wish all of what I went through in dealing with Patrick's illness and death never happened, but it brought me experiences I never would have known if I hadn't been open to it.

I never would have been able to deal with my own illness without them.

I learned to look beyond the loss, hurt, and pain, and to reach out and touch. Touch heals as it comforts.

Face your fear, anger, and pain. You have to work through it and not get stuck. If you don't, you may not be whole; you may survive but remain bitter and angry.

You have no time to be bitter and angry.

Those feelings limit your abilities. You have to work through them. An angry life is an empty life. It prevents you from experiencing compassion, love, and gentleness. You have to be kind to yourself when you are hurting.

When I was recovering from my surgery and chemo, so many people said to me, "How did you do it? You were so strong."

I really wasn't.

They just didn't always see me.

This was another thing I learned. People are not that observant. They are not always in tune. Maybe it's a coping mechanism for them.

Maybe it's a sign of the times. We are in such a rush that we don't take in everything along the way.

So many people never even noticed my unbalanced gait. They never saw that I was in pain. But there were those who did.

Maybe I got good at being observant because the one thing I had when I was sick was time to do things, but I was too weak to really do much of anything but observe.

I never did this before — sit still, think, and observe, but cancer taught me that lesson because I was so fatigued all the time.

When I was recovering from a virus, I was so weak that there were times when all I could do was go from the chair to the couch to the bed.

At each stop along the way, I dozed off. But I could sit in the living room and look out the windows and notice things I never saw before, like branches, the same branches that were there for years, but I noticed the character they had and wondered about the intricacies of them, and how special that was.

There was a bird that I named because I swear he was looking at me in my stillness as I was looking at him. We really connected, and when he came by, I was happy to see him. Every day I looked for him, waited and wondered if he would come.

He moved from the tree branch to the garage roof over to the holly bush. It was funny, because that year our holly bush was so full of berries, and I watched the birds eat them off the bush. It was amazing how much they ate. I would've never seen this if cancer hadn't forced me to slow down and just be.

Anger and fear make for a lonely life. They cause you to slowly remove people from your life and replace them with negative emotions.

That is a high price to pay just to stay angry.

So I consciously decided no anger. What's the point? Did I get frustrated? You bet I did. Was I upset? Yes, but I tried not to let it turn into anger, and I tried hard to deal with my feelings so I could get through it.

One time I got very angry, but I felt impatient more than anything else. I was in the hospital, and Jimmy kept asking me questions in his efforts to help: Did I want this? What to do about that? Could he do this for me?

I think I wanted him to just be and accept this juncture in our lives, and stop asking me questions. The last thing I wanted was to be asked questions.

I was thinking, *If you really wanted to do something you would just do it and let it be done*. I snapped at him, and it really upset him, which upset me and everybody else in the room. He had no idea why I was upset, and maybe I didn't either, but nonetheless, we had this episode to deal with, and we did.

Which brings us to the fact that with illness comes stress.

When my brother was sick and in the hospital, there was a lot to be done, coordinated, and tended to. Sometimes there were stressful situations between Patrick and me.

I guess what I realized from the very beginning of my illness was that Jimmy and I were going to have a role reversal.

When my husband turned fifty, he was diagnosed with cancer. He took it all in stride, so it appeared. Me? I was fraught with worry. That's what a spouse does: you worry about the what-ifs. You keep a watchful eye for the next change, the next shoe to drop. As the spouse/caregiver, you control nothing.

When I became the patient, I learned that it's so much easier to be the patient. The patient knows how they feel; there is nothing to imagine. As the patient, you know the plan and where you are going, and you take things as they come.

The spouse/caregiver does not have that luxury. This was the hardest thing for me to contemplate because I knew the journey my husband was about to be on. I was so upset; I would do anything to spare him from what I had gone through when I was his caregiver. So many times I felt that the surgery or chemo was grueling, but I was caring for me now, not a family, holding up the rear and bracing for whatever was coming.

As bad as it is for the patient, it is ten times worse for the spouse/caregiver. Now we had to go through this together. We had come full circle!

Whether connections or coincidences, my life has had a series of lessons that have prepared me to deal with my illness and Jimmy's. This didn't make it easy, but I was able to focus on the healing process and all its components. Much has been written and stated about our healthcare system, but it is only when you are embedded in it that you can appreciate its complexity.

Health care is not only comprised of hospitals, pharmaceuticals, and insurers. All of these are extremely important, but what is vital to successful outcomes are the women and men who deliver healthcare to patients, and the families and friends who provide their after care.

Jimmy and I have been blessed. We have had the best of both worlds. Our medical team has been first rate. Our family and friends are the best.

They all have given us the reason and ability to live well.

The Genius Of Kids

I don't think I was one of those fathers who talked incessantly about his kids. I don't think I ever whipped out a family album of pictures from my wallet to show off their cuteness. So, I think I can be indulged to relate their early demonstrations of genius.

When Sean was born, Eileen and I lived in New Rochelle. She worked evenings in a local hospital, and I taught in a Catholic high school in the Bronx. Eileen left for work at about three in the afternoon, and one of our terrific neighbors watched Sean for a few hours before I got home.

One evening, I had finished feeding Sean, and he was even bathed and ready for bed. He could only have been about four months old. He was sitting on the floor in one of those little seats, and I was sitting on the floor next to him.

After a few minutes, I thought it was time to give him his bottle and get him in the mood for a good night's sleep, so I got up from the floor. Well, I attempted to get up, and stumbled while doing so.

Sean laughed out loud at my mishap, a true belly laugh. At this tender age, he got slapstick and showed his appreciation at my attempt to amuse. Of course, he might have been laughing at the notion that I was the adult in charge of his welfare, and I could barely take care of myself.

I was stunned that Sean had already developed a sense of humor.

A few years later, it was Jeannine's turn to amaze.

She was two or three years old, and we were sitting at opposite ends of the couch. I looked at her and said how beautiful she was, to which she replied, "Do you really mean that?"

Maybe I'm easy to stun, but here again, I was amazed that this little girl understood that people were often disingenuous. She still believed in Santa Claus (as do I, by the way), but she had already figured out that men bullshit women all the time.

I always used to say that Jeannine was my barometer. She always was able to identify a jerk, and likewise, was able to discern a pure, noble creature.

Bryan cannot be excluded from this tale.

There are two stories I will tell of Bryan. The first occurred when he was two or three. Eileen was working, and I was in charge. I had prepared a meal for Bryan consisting of rice with chicken neatly diced into small pieces. I tasted it myself, and it was quite good. It wasn't baby food out of a jar. I had done the preparations and cooking.

To encourage his eating this excellent meal, I positioned his high chair in such a way that he could see the television and watch his favorite show, *Thomas the Tank Engine*. (I know, I'm a terrible father, but it was PBS, and Ringo Starr was Mr. Conductor that day, so give me a break.)

Watching Bryan pick at his meal, I endeavored to up the ante and put three small chocolate chip cookies on the counter adjacent to his high chair.

"Now, Bryan, if you eat your dinner, you can have those cookies."

He continued to pick but not with the gusto I had hoped for.

Once more, I admonished Bryan and encouraged him to finish his meal.

Finally, in exasperation at his continued slow-motion attempt to not eat his food I said, "Do you want me to eat those cookies?"

To which he replied, "No, I want you to eat my chicken."

I gave up.

I am not sure how much time had gone by since the chicken incident, but another Saturday had come, and Eileen was working. This time I was in charge of starting Bryan's potty training program.

There would be no diaper worn today, only little boy underwear.

Bryan was an eager and attentive student. When the first moment came, he ran into the bathroom with me a few feet behind to offer any needed assistance.

I saw Bryan deftly lower his underwear, and then, in a highly exasperated tone, as he lifted the toilet seat, he uttered this pearl of wisdom:

"People who sit should leave the seat up for people who stand."

Oh, my God!

Why is the man always in charge of the seat?

Why can't women be considerate and leave the seat up for us?

I get that it's not politically correct to start this debate, but Bryan uttered a notion that all men surely have thought at some point in their lives.

Those are just a few of the reasons that Sean, Jeannine, and Bryan have brought so much joy to Eileen and me. The next three essays only add to our pride and joy.

We thought it would be insightful to allow our children to describe what it was like for them to witness what Eileen and I went through as we dealt with cancer. Although the title of our book is *Married With Cancer*, this disease strikes all who have to watch their loved ones struggle with this beast.

Sean, Jeannine, and Bryan offer their unique perspectives and will certainly support and challenge much of what we have written. We will be reminded, once again, that caregivers bear a special burden on the journey of survival.

Sean will be the first to offer his perspective.

Sean

When I first heard that Dad had leukemia, my initial, off-the-cuff reaction was a mixture of anger and disbelief. I had just come back from a trip to Philly with all my friends, and you guys said you decided to hold off on telling me until I got back so it wouldn't ruin the trip.

I know why you did that, but this was my dad, and cancer! I got over my initial anger and frustration, and my feelings switched to concern and fear. I specifically remember thinking about having to give a eulogy and what I would say — and then those feelings soon gave way to the emotional equivalent of a sort of dull, nagging pain that was just always there.

Dad was always good about downplaying it, and for the most part, that put me at ease. It was still difficult to see the toll it took on him, even as infrequently as I did, since I was away at college.

Being away was good and bad. I felt cut off, but I also had my friends to retreat to. Khalil and I formed a bond as we both struggled with the mortality of our fathers. And, honestly, cutting myself off is what I do in these types of situations.

For instance, I never went to see Uncle Michael in the hospital. I still don't honestly know if I regret that or not. I regret not being able to say goodbye, but I don't regret not *having* to say goodbye, seeing him like that, if that makes sense. I don't regret not knowing what he looked like in the hospital.

Mom was different. She would show cracks every now and then when Dad was sick, but I never saw her falter once when she got sick, which made it harder because I knew she was lying. I also didn't have my support system around when she was sick like I did when Dad got sick. I was physically cut off from all my close friends, going through whatever I was going through with my girlfriend at the time. I hated my job, and that caused me a lot of stress, and now Parent No. 2 had just been tagged with the Big C. It didn't register at the time, but I have to admit that selfishly, it was a dark period in my life.

Dad's hair grayed and thinned a little during his chemo treatments, but the changes were much more visible when Mom went through hers. The loss of strength she suffered and the fight she put up sapped her of her personality and liveliness, and it felt like cancer took my mom away for a long time.

It's a crazy feeling to realize that and actually put it into words. I know it didn't happen overnight like this, but I also have a specific memory of being back at the house and Mom bustling around trying to get us to tidy up before someone came over to visit, and that's when I knew she was back.

Jeannine

Ten years and countless other variables separate the experiences of both my parents having cancer.

I was sixteen years old when my dad was diagnosed with CLL, and ten years later, my mom was diagnosed with breast cancer.

When I found out that Dad had CLL, I was devastated. I had just returned from a trip to Ireland with my Aunt Mary. Mom and Dad had actually gotten the news before I left, but they knew better than to share that with me and then send me off to a foreign country.

At the time, I was mad that they waited and held that information from me, but now that I'm an adult, I understand. I was a sophomore in high school, a late bloomer who was just starting to come into her own.

While I felt very compassionate for what my dad was about to go through, and for what our family would experience alongside him, my egocentric teenage brain focused mostly on myself: Why is this awful thing happening to *me* and *my* family?

How is this going to affect *my* life?

What will *I* do if my dad dies?

Dad, being the perpetual funny-man, did not allow himself or anyone else to wallow in their feelings. He wanted everything to be normal. He did, however, get exceptionally good at the Irish Guilt Trip. He would say things like, "Could you go get a beer for your father who has cancer?" and "You're really going out to spend time with your friends when your father is at home with cancer?"

I don't think he knew this at the time, but those comments were really hard on me. I understood that he was trying to make light of the situation, but I couldn't help but feel there was some truth to his statements, and the guilt that followed was very real.

Naturally, over the course of the next ten years, I grew up, went to college, moved out on my own, and started working as a teacher. The story of my mom's cancer diagnosis is a very interesting one.

It was summertime, July, I believe. I had just spent a few days in Boston because I was contemplating moving there. While I was in Boston, I met some potential roommates and looked at an apartment with them. I also had a very promising job interview with Cambridge Public Schools. As I took the ferry back home to East Quogue, I weighed the pros and cons of moving from the Bronx to Boston.

There were very few cons, although I knew I would miss being so close to my family if I moved. I was so excited to share this news with my parents and hear their thoughts about what I should do.

I arrived home in the early afternoon before anyone was home from work. For some reason, I decided to check the answering machine, even though I never received calls at my parents' house. A few mundane messages played, and then I heard Aunt Pat's voice on the machine. She didn't sound like her normal chipper self. I don't really remember what she said (something about a doctor's visit, or a test), but by the end of that message, I knew that something very serious was going on with my mom.

I sat with that information for a few hours, waiting for my mom to return home from work. It was a blessing, really, because it allowed me to prepare. It still wasn't easy to hear what my mom had to say, but I was ready for it.

And then came the decision: to move or not to move? At the time, it felt like the hardest decision of my life, but thinking back on it now, it seems obvious that there was no choice. There is no way I could have left my mom and family at the end of that summer. That was the first adult decision I made, and I never looked back.

The treatments that Mom and Dad received were very different, but in some ways, they rendered the same fears: What if this doesn't work? How will this change their quality of life? What if this kills them before the cancer does?

I remember accompanying Dad to one of his treatments. We were in the Riverhead office, and I think it was snowing. The nurse came to check on him and brought him a blanket. At that point, I realized that he was shaking.

I asked if he was okay, and he referred to this as "the rigors." He said that it happens sometimes, and it was nothing to worry about. But to watch my dad sit in a chair, hooked up to an IV, and shake uncontrollably through his treatment was not an easy sight to bear.

It was a reminder of the fragility of cancer patients, the fragility of my dad — and it brought back all of those fears and worries you try to keep in the back of your mind so as not to go down the rabbit hole on endless what-if scenarios.

Unfortunately, Mom suffered many more experiences like this throughout her treatment period.

Whether it was peeling off layers of skin from the soles of her feet, losing her hair, or having to pause her treatment to give her body a chance to recover, all of these highlighted just how terrible cancer treatment could be.

When I found out that my mom was sick, I didn't think about myself the way I had when Dad was initially diagnosed. I think this is where the age difference really comes into play. Maturity and responsibility forced me to focus on my mom above anyone else, and after that, I focused on my family.

That allowed me to be present and aware of what was going on in ways that I hadn't with my dad. Everything with my dad's cancer was "escape" or "deny," but with my mom, there was no escaping. After her surgery, she taught me how to empty and measure her drains and replace the bandages.

I tried to make sure that the house was kept clean (and if not clean, at least neat), and there was food in the house. I made sure to visit frequently and accompany her to treatments whenever possible. When she got vertigo, my dad and I had to walk her to the bathroom and back, and help her in and out of bed. When she wound up in the hospital for a few days, everyone was on edge. The fear of the unknown was palpable. Like I said, there was no escaping when Mom was sick.

The greatest lesson from Dad's cancer was easy to identify: life is short and unpredictable, so you have to do the things that matter.

For us, this meant taking vacations, building an addition onto the house, and for me, taking a drive out to East Quogue for the day, or even just to have lunch — showing up when it wasn't always easy or ideal, and taking care of one another.

In short, you could reduce this all to the notion of time. We never seem to have enough of it, but when something matters a great deal, you somehow manage to find the time, and that is a gift.

The greatest lesson from Mom's cancer is a little more complicated. Having both parents experience a life-threatening illness can be very taxing on family dynamics. We watched my mom, a nurse and the perpetual caretaker, become the patient, and my dad, who was still a patient himself, assume the role of caretaker. And because so much time had passed between their diagnoses, we were all different people by the time my mom got sick, and the roles we played during my dad's illness were not necessarily the roles we played during my mom's.

I guess the lesson here is that people can only do what they can do, and chances are, they're doing the best they can. And that has to be okay.

Of course, difficult or negative feelings may arise because of these shifts in family dynamics, but ultimately, you have to reach the point of understanding that we're all doing the best we can. When I was able to look at it from that perspective, it helped dissipate any feelings of anger or resentment that had been lingering. It allowed me to move toward acceptance and forgiveness.

Bryan

When I found out my dad had leukemia, I didn't really know what to make of it. I was in fifth grade, and I remember knowing that it meant he was sick, but that he was going to be okay.

Growing up, Dad and I watched a lot of sports and went to many a Yankee game. I've got so many great memories of going to games with him. I remember going to a Yankee-Red Sox game with him and Uncle Vinnie.

I remember Dad missing a monster home run from Darryl Strawberry (one of my favorites growing up) because I had to go to the bathroom or wanted a hot dog or something typical that kids do.

I remember the feeling of Yankee Stadium literally shaking beneath my feet when David Justice and Bernie Williams combined for back-to-back (and belly-to-belly) home runs to tie and then win the game in walk-off fashion.

I remember Sean being at the game Jeter hit his one and only Grand Slam, and I remember him catching a home run ball that was hit by someone on the White Sox team during batting practice before a playoff game.

I remember Dad getting two tickets to the last game at the old Yankee Stadium and insisting that Sean and I go. We saw Val Kilmer, Spike Lee, and Reggie Jackson at that game.

We were sitting near where Reggie hit his third home run in Game 6 against the Dodgers, cementing himself as Mr. October forever. (We were actually at the stadium with Dad when Mike Stanley had his own three-homer day.)

Spike Lee had brought Reggie up there to talk about that night — just one of the many memorable Yankee moments that took place on that hallowed ground that was about to shut its doors for good. I remember sneaking down to the sideline in right field with Sean later that night so we could scoop up some dirt to take home.

But one of our favorite stories in the Newell household is about a seminal Yankees moment that we *almost* saw in person.

On a lark, Dad decided one morning that we should drive in and see a Yankee game because it was Yogi Berra Day. We got off to a bit of a late start, though, and when we hadn't left by eleven in the morning, Dad decided not to go in. He probably thought we wouldn't get there in time for Yogi's ceremony, not to mention we didn't have tickets, it was a Sunday, and Dad had work the next day. We honestly didn't think anything of it at the time. But when we sat down to watch the game on TV, we realized too late that we had missed out on witnessing history. David Cone threw a perfect game that day, and Dad's been kicking himself ever since.

This was before his diagnosis, but looking back, he's wondered if maybe this was an early sign, because if you know Jim Newell, you know that a late start is a rarity, an anomaly, a phenomenon.

This is a man who gets to the airport four hours early. And so he wonders if he was feeling fatigued that day, and thinks maybe that was a bit of foreshadowing for the diagnosis to come.

I hope he doesn't feel like we missed out on something that day, or that it was somehow his fault. I'm sure we had a great afternoon at home. We probably grilled up some dogs and then laughed at ourselves in bemusement as the game unfolded. I hope he doesn't blame himself for "missing out" on that day, on that one memory, because there were so many others over the years that this one doesn't sting.

Besides, the thing at the center of those memories wasn't what happened on the field. It was about being there and sharing those moments together, even if the moment was waiting in line for a hot dog and only hearing the reaction to a home run instead of seeing it for ourselves.

And for the record, I eventually did get to see a perfect game in person, only it was a Boston Red Sox game pitched by Jon Lester at Fenway Park, so it's not as much fun to talk about.

Mom's cancer diagnosis is another story.

Dad's cancer was a cakewalk in comparison.

I found out about Mom's diagnosis on a Skype call while in London for a five-week study abroad program. The call started just like you'd expect, a "Hey-how's-London-we're-just-catching-up-we-miss-you" call from your parents while you're across the Atlantic for the first time.

Then the atmosphere or tone of the call changed. They said they had some bad news. My immediate reaction was, "Oh, shit, I know I paid off that open container ticket I got from the NYPD over spring break weekend, but maybe they found out somehow." For the record, they've never known about this ticket and are learning of it now for the first time!

But then I got the *actual* bad news. Mom had breast cancer, and she needed surgery and then chemotherapy and radiation.

I still had a month to go in the study abroad program. Mom and Dad told me they didn't want me to come back home unless I wanted to, and that they held off on telling me because they wanted me to have this study abroad experience. I don't think there's anything else I can say beyond that to sum up the generosity, kindness, and sacrifice that my mother embodies, but I'll try.

The news shook me. I debated going back home. It may have been a few days after I got the news, but I'll never forget sitting down on a small stone bench in a garden and crying.

I was on my way to print a paper that I'd been up all night writing, so I was already a little sleep deprived. That's when the appropriately titled "Far" by Coheed and Cambria started playing through my headphones. And I just wept.

It isn't the best song ever, and it comes off my least favorite album of theirs and one I rarely re-visit, but the sentiment of being far away struck a chord. It didn't help that before I left for my trip, that same album was playing just before Mom and I got into a little bit of a fight over something stupid that I can't even remember at this point, something that was probably my fault.

Regretting that fight, missing my mom, feeling scared about what might happen — it all just collided as that song played, and there was nothing for it but to sit down and let it out.

I think what felt different about Mom's diagnosis was that she was always so steady in our lives. Dad did a good job of downplaying his leukemia, and he was so good at making a joke out of it that it never felt all that serious.

Also, I was much younger when he was diagnosed, and so the whole thing, at least at first, was a little over my head, and Mom was always there if we needed to talk about Dad. She did her best to make sure that things went on as normally as possible for us.

To see her strength in those moments be rewarded with her own cancer diagnosis was the very definition of unfair. We already felt so blessed that Dad had gotten through his treatments and entered remission. It just didn't feel like we'd get that lucky again.

Somehow, we did.

Jimmy and Eileen

You can see how we were able to get through our ordeal. When you have three exceptional children as sensitive and strong as Sean, Jeannine, and Bryan are, you cannot help but feel blessed.

Each is different in his or her way, but they share a common spirit, joy, and compassion, which was so powerful and instrumental in our recovery.

Their sense of humor never faltered, and as tough as those times really were, we have many memories of laughter around the dinner table or when playing the family favorite card game "May I."

Sean, Jeannine, and Bryan remain our source of strength and wellbeing.

There are good things that come from cancer, gifts that perhaps others do not get to experience, such as sharing and facing the frightening reality of the unknown. Because of cancer, we were all able to grow in ways we never thought possible.

You really don't prepare your children to deal with cancer because you don't anticipate that they will have to.

In order to do this well and prepare your family as you prepare yourself, you need to be present.

Being present doesn't mean you need to like your situation, but it does mean that when you acknowledge what you're going through, you include others and make a plan where you previously may not have done so.

Our struggle with cancer provided cherished memories and made each of us grow, and it brought our family closer together.

Cancer has, no doubt, helped to shape our ability to respond to whatever challenges await us.

We are so grateful for this part of our life.

Gratitude

We live in a material world. As such, I often find myself focusing on the things I have and the things I don't yet have but want. Jimmy is often worse than me because he just loves going on eBay to bid on Lionel trains.

The reality is that neither of us is ever satisfied with the things we buy. What we really treasure is that we still have each other even after cancer.

What possession could ever compete with that?

Not only do we still have each other, we have our three beautiful children and their dogs!

Jimmy and I now live in Florida, and it has been an adjustment leaving our children behind, but they have been down several times to visit, and we have returned to New York a few times to visit them.

When we told our children that we were selling the house in East Quogue, Jimmy said, "We are selling our house, not our home. Our home will be Florida, and it will always be your home too."

In the dark days when I was going through chemo and didn't really know if I would survive, I never lost gratitude for my family.

In many ways, I think gratitude was as powerful in defeating my cancer as any of the treatments I endured. When we work at making ourselves better, we make things better in the world.

My gratitude was not just for my children and husband but my entire family. My sister Mary, my brothers Jimmy and Kevin, all helped me during that terrible year.

Then there are my friends.

Pat Lowenwirth

Pat Darcey

Connie Andersen

Karen DeSimone

You've read about them already. You know how they helped me survive. My heartfelt wish for you is that you have friends like this wonderful group of mine.

Jimmy has said several times over the years that he doesn't want to take his remission for granted. He usually says this when he is starting a diet.

We remind ourselves from time to time about the miracle that we have both experienced. To be able to go to sleep in the same bed and get up to share a breakfast together is perhaps the most significant miracle of all.

It's something I never take for granted, and it is just one of the many, many things for which I feel such a sense of gratitude.

Gratitude is my after-care plan. It continues to keep me well.

Our Night With A Knight

Late one night in the middle of November 1963, a night that would soon change to early one morning, I heard a song on my Dick Tracy transistor radio that would change my life forever. I heard it once around midnight, and I couldn't go to sleep until I heard it again. The song was "I Want To Hold Your Hand" by a group from England of all places.

Well, I wasn't the only one who heard that song as the Beatles came roaring into our lives. You might say they saved our lives. I always thought that their first hit, my all-time favorite song that I heard back on that night in 1963, was exactly what the country needed just a few weeks after I first heard it.

In the dark days that followed when we were sucker punched by Lee Harvey Oswald, we needed someone to hold our collective hands, and the Beatles showed up just in the nick of time. The trouble was not everyone "got" the Beatles. Some ridiculed their look. Others denied their harmony and musical talent.

This is how I was introduced to the world of the iconic Sixties. It took a few years for it all to sink in, but my worldview was altered forever.

All these emotions presented themselves to me the night that I sat in the upper deck of Yankee Stadium with my family for Eileen's coming out party, as she liked to describe it. (She was one year removed from breast cancer and surgery.) There I was in the Bronx where forty-eight years ago, I first heard "I Want To Hold Your Hand" while lying in my bed at 1261 Leland Avenue, but on this momentous occasion, I was waiting for Paul McCartney to take the stage. When he finally did, I was overwhelmed. I didn't know whether to laugh or cry. Fortunately, I did neither, but I must have had a quizzical look on my face because Eileen kept asking me if I was all right.

Paul, or as I like to refer to him, Sir Paul, started singing around 8:30 p.m., and didn't leave the stage till around 11:20. All-time great songs just rolled along one after another: "Hello Goodbye," "Eleanor Rigby," "Jet," and perhaps the shocker of them all, "A Day In A Life." I tried to take videos of all the songs, and every time he went to the piano, I just knew he was going to sing "Hey Jude." But, as luck would have it, that did not come until the end of the show, and as I started my video, that sick little twirling spiral indicating that my iPhone was shutting down appeared on my screen. *Oh well,* I thought, *I'll get it the next night on our second night with a knight.*

I am frequently lovingly kidded about my online shopping tendencies, mostly on eBay but sometimes on other sites. I book Disney vacations and pay for Yankee tickets online, but for this momentous occasion, I called Eileen for permission to make my purchase.

Calling Eileen at work was often a pointless endeavor. One meeting after another or some other Joint Commission emergency kept her away from her desk at Southampton Hospital. This day, however, she picked up on the first ring.

I told her Paul McCartney was playing at Yankee Stadium and asked her if she thought I should try to get tickets. She didn't hesitate and told me to get tickets for our kids as well.

Several hundred dollars later, I called to confirm that we would be attending the Friday night show. She then confided that she wanted our friends Pat and Paul to come with us. I told her that there was another show the next night, and she said, "Get off the phone and get the tickets!"

I did as directed, and now Eileen and I were going to see Sir Paul two nights in a row.

I could tell this was very special for Eileen. Almost a year prior to the day we made our way to see a Beatle, she had sat me down to tell me she had breast cancer, and her prognosis did not look good.

Surgery, chemo, and radiation interspersed with terrible reactions to the entire ordeal, not to mention shaving her head before she started chemo, made the prospect of our attending this concert with a healthy Eileen just another miracle along the journey.

Eileen's hair was starting to grow back, and she looked absolutely gorgeous as we sat in our seats in the upper deck of Yankee Stadium.

Eileen had her own feelings on the subject.

"When you are going through your treatment plan, it is a good idea to have a goal. During my treatment recovery, I heard that Paul McCartney was going to be doing a concert in New York City in a few months. It became my goal to be well enough to go, to be able to walk the long distance from the parking lot to the venue, and to reach my seat independently. It made me happy to think about it and kept me focused on the goal. You need that to keep yourself going. We went. In fact, we went twice. It was incredible!"

The concert was magnificent and memorable in so many ways, but the wonder of the night was sitting next to Eileen and seeing the joy in her face and the smile that had won my heart forty years earlier.

Emotionally Yours

I think the commonality that Eileen and I have shared during our journey with cancer is that we have acknowledged our emotions.

Laughing at yourself and each other is okay. We did our share of crying too.

When Eileen was sick and had her head shaved, the entire family did not cry or exhibit any tendency that we were in a grave situation. We laughed and even quoted a favorite *Seinfeld* episode where George wears a wig on a blind date with a woman who he doesn't realize is bald until he meets her for the first time.

"She's bald, Jerry. She's bald! She's BALD!"

Eileen was never one to let things get to her, and she laughed along with us.

Later that evening, she donned a kerchief on her head, and we were all given kerchiefs to wear as we played our favorite card game, "May I."

Although we knew the severe nature of the battle she was beginning, we also knew that she was a worthy opponent, and she would prevail.

We couldn't bring ourselves to consider any other possibility.

Laughter was always part of our arsenal while fighting this dreaded disease, but there was crying too. More often the crying was brought on by the miracle of the life that continued.

I found myself crying at the drop of a hat.

Every year in early December, Fordham University presents Lessons and Carols on the Bronx campus. We first started to attend this event when Jeannine was a student at Fordham.

We didn't get there every year, but we did attend in 2011 when Eileen was getting back to normal. Her hair had almost entirely grown back by then, and she looked as beautiful as ever.

Lessons and Carols consisted of various Fordham University glee clubs and choirs singing traditional hymns and carols interspersed with biblical readings recited by students and Jesuit priests. For Eileen and me, there is no better way to begin the holidays in earnest.

But then there's the crying.

Each year the students sing "Once in Royal David's City," and I am not sure if it is the words or the ethereal nature of the music, but I immediately go into blubber mode. Eileen has to hold my hand to prevent me from going into an all-out weeping accompaniment drowning out singers and pipe organ.

I soon recovered and enjoyed the remaining songs and readings. Of course, I endured some severe kidding about my weepiness when we went out for dinner later in the evening.

But crying isn't the only emotion I succumb to.

I have been known to enter a trance or to experience a deep sense of awe and wonder while I am at Yankee Stadium.

On one occasion, when I was at a game with Bryan, it was the ninth inning, and Metallica's "Enter Sandman" was blasting on the stadium PA system. The reason for this particular song was that Mariano Rivera, the best closer in baseball history, was entering the game.

If you are not a baseball fan, you can put the book down for a minute and Google Mariano Rivera so that you can understand the following story.

As the song blared and Mariano jogged toward the pitcher's mound, I turned to Bryan and said, "Do you get this?" He looked at me blankly and shook his head like he didn't get my drift, so I said it again, and finally, he replied in a rather miffed tone, "Yeah, I get it!"

I am not sure he understood the portent behind my question. The moment the music started, I thought of my father.

He was a primary reason why I was raised a Yankee fan. He grew up in the age of Babe Ruth and Lou Gherig, and told me all about them as well as Joe DiMaggio. He loved Mickey Mantle as I had learned to. Here I was with Bryan thinking how great it would have been to be with Pop to see Babe Ruth hit a homer. How great would it have been to see Lou Gherig crush a ball into the stands with my father at my side?

Here I was with my son witnessing the best, the absolute best, the Babe Ruth of closers jog onto the field and get the final three outs of another Yankee victory. Perhaps dealing with cancer helped me appreciate life more than I had before. I no longer took Eileen for granted nor my children nor my friends. I also never took these special moments for granted, moments that are fleeting and often never experienced again.

Separate But Unequal

Despite having a beautiful great room with a big fireplace, I often spent my free time downstairs in what I referred to as my TV room. Our finished basement, compliments of Eileen's brother Jimmy, served as my man cave.

It was equipped with dozens and dozens (I am afraid to say hundreds and hundreds) of Lionel trains, my MAC computer, and my 70-inch high-def TV thanks to our dear friend Karen DeSimone.

It was where I went to get away from it all.

I watched the New York Yankees when I was not at Yankee Stadium on Saturdays. I watched the New York Jets when I was not at Met Life Stadium. I watched the New York Rangers for whom I couldn't afford season tickets.

It was where I vegged out after chemo treatments.

It was where I went early on Saturday mornings to watch *The Adventures of Superman* on DVD.

Eileen didn't mind. When the kids were home, she and Jeannine watched shows that I definitely didn't want to watch. There was only a 32-inch TV in the living room, but Eileen was okay with that. She didn't need a big screen or surround sound.

Then she got sick.

By this time, everyone was out of the house. Sean was working and living in the Bronx. Jeannine had finished her masters and was teaching and living in the Bronx. Bryan was in his last year at Fordham University, also in the Bronx.

Because of this, my TV habits changed.

I couldn't go downstairs to my man cave and leave Eileen alone upstairs. How could I? I have been known to be selfish at times, but I am not that bad, and having experienced the fright that I might lose her, I just couldn't do it.

So Eileen and I sat on the sofa and watched whatever she wanted to watch. We soon realized that the one type of show that we both enjoyed was cooking shows. We were fortunate because our cable package included the cooking channels, and the local public broadcasting channel had many cooking shows that we just loved.

We loved to watch Lidia Bastianich prepare delicious Italian meals. Then there was *America's Test Kitchen*, which, in addition to cooking two scrumptious-looking meals, had segments on food tasting and equipment testing. These were my favorite, and I often went straight to my iPad to order whatever they had just reviewed.

We still watch these shows down in Florida as well as one of my all-time favorites, *Nick Stellino: Storyteller in the Kitchen*.

These shows not only entertained me, but they inspired me to get into cooking. I have a sneaky suspicion that Eileen had that in mind when she introduced me to these shows.

So, we would head out on a Saturday morning to the local farmers' market and specialty shops to purchase that weekend's ingredients for our Saturday and Sunday feasts, including fresh pasta and everything needed for her bolognese sauce, and chicken cutlets for her chicken francaise.

Then I would visit our local beer distributor to purchase Blue Point Hoptical Illusion, a local Long Island craft beer just because I needed something to sip by the fire.

These moments of shopping and cooking together added joy to our life, and it was an opportunity for me to develop new cooking skills. Now, to be fair, I was more of a sous chef than a real chef. I didn't make the bolognese sauce as much as open the cans of tomatoes. I did get to clean the chicken cutlets, and sometimes I chopped vegetables to the extent that I got them out of the refrigerator.

I have "Jimmy" hands and really can't be trusted with sharp knives or fragile cookware for that matter. When dicing and chopping had to be done, I was ordered to leave the kitchen. It was the Jimmy hands, and she didn't want to expose me to danger. This continues to be a running joke, and as with most jokes, there is quite a bit of truth to the humor.

Regardless of my diminished role in the kitchen, we had fun preparing our meals knowing that we would have a delicious dinner to share with our guests.

I've always been able to step out of a situation and observe what is going on as if I'm not there, as if I'm watching a movie. I did this all the time when I was a kid at a particularly enjoyable party and more often as an adult at a family Christmas party or some other special gathering of family and friends. So, it was often common for me to step back and appreciate the miracle of Eileen working in the kitchen. She was so intent in her preparations, and it was a miracle to realize that she was still here with me, and that it might not have been that way, but thank God it was, and she was still here exasperated with the mess I leave in the kitchen when I make my mother's Irish soda bread.

Living The Good Life

As you might imagine, any two people dealing with a severe situation are likely to have different approaches as to how to cope. Not surprising to me, Eileen and I were in full agreement with the way each of us dealt with cancer.

Cancer was not going to define who we were. I had moments when I not only refused to think of myself as a cancer survivor, but I questioned whether I ever had CLL in the first place.

Fortunately, I had many years when I never felt ill. I was able to go to work and rarely had any health issues to deal with. Eileen, for her part, refused to identify as a breast cancer survivor. God forbid you were to get her a pink Yankee hat! It wasn't that she was insensitive to her fellow breast cancer survivors, but she didn't want that to be her identity.

This mindset of putting cancer behind us did not result in a reckless approach to our health, as we both continued our regular check-ups, and anytime I happened to have a sniffle, my live-in nurse would be after me to listen to my body and stay home. Eileen also made sure that we ate healthy, but more importantly, lived a good life.

It seemed that I had just finished my first battery of chemo when she started talking about renovating our house in East

Quogue. The plan was that we would add a dining room to give us extra space for entertaining. Despite the fact that I observed that our house was big enough to host our very large extended family's annual Christmas party, she convinced me that we needed more room.

This was in 2004.

Sean had graduated from college and was in the middle of law school.

Jeannine was a sophomore in college soon to be entering her junior year.

Bryan was the only child still living at home, and in three short years, he would be off to college.

Because of this, I didn't think we needed to make our house bigger because our family was shrinking.

Nevertheless, we proceeded and talked to a contractor.

The first contractor gave us a plan and a cost estimate of about fifty thousand dollars. We thought that was reasonable and were about to sign the deal. The one snag in the process was that this particular contractor seemed to have disappeared off the face of the earth. So, that plan was nixed before it ever got started.

Eileen's brother Jimmy suggested we consult a local contractor who had an office right around the corner from us, so Eileen called and made an appointment. Unfortunately, the appointment was made for the day of the St. Patrick's Day parade in Westhampton. I just had to go to the parade, so I let Eileen meet with the contractor.

Big mistake.

I came home from the parade, and before I knew it, the fifty thousand dollar project had grown to two hundred thousand. Now, I must admit that I had as much to do with this as anyone. However, before I had even come home the simple plan of adding a dining room was replaced by adding a new kitchen to complement the dining room. Then we got talking.

Raising a family in a house with only one bathroom was often a challenge. Then, too, selling a house with only one bathroom might also prove to be problematic. Not that we were planning to move anytime soon, but you do have to think about the future.

A bathroom was added to the project.

Now, I really don't remember how the great room made it to the blueprints, but there it was, and then I asked, "Where's the fireplace?"

You see, we had a fireplace in our old living room, but now the living room was going to be the dining room. So, while it would be nice to have a crackling fire when you are having Thanksgiving dinner or Christmas dinner, sitting in the dining room on a cold Saturday evening would not cut it.

I needed a fireplace in the great room.

Construction began in July 2004, and the first order of business was the demolition of our mudroom and deck and outdoor shower. When I saw that the excavation plan included the destruction of the pipe connection to our cesspool, I almost fainted.

You see, the next day I was to have a colonoscopy, and I had to do the dreaded prep cocktail that afternoon.

I went out and frantically appealed to the contractor and his men. They all had a good laugh at my expense as they directed me to the port-o-potty in the front yard. After five minutes of this good-natured kidding, they assured me that I would be "good to go" by three that afternoon.

By October the project was completed, and the first Saturday after the completion, Eileen and I walked around to the contractor's office. Eileen had a speech prepared which she hadn't shared with me.

She let these big burly men know that their skill and hard work were so appreciated. She let them know that only three years ago I was in chemotherapy. The project that may have started out as an architect's sketch and a pile of wood and other building materials had recreated a life that was in need of being put back together.

To Eileen, this renovation was not only my resurrection; it represented our future together.

Our construction crew took turns hugging Eileen and me right in their office. They had tears in their eyes. What a gift Eileen had given them. Their work was so much more than a renovation, and you could see how sincerely they appreciated Eileen's emotional tribute. The only thing Eileen didn't realize was that she would spend more than a year living in the beautiful room going from couch to chair and taking in all that nature had to offer outside its windows.

As if being guided by other forces, Eileen's desire to redesign our house also served to sustain her when the time came for her to battle cancer six years later.

In February 2010, a short five months before Eileen's diagnosis, we had a snow day and were both at home from work. Now, that didn't stop us from going to a favorite store in Southampton to purchase a considerable L-shaped sofa.

This sofa had a sofa bed, which came in very handy. It also had three couches that could accommodate three nurses napping — Eileen, Connie, and Karen.

When Eileen had her surgery, Connie and Karen stayed a week to care for her, and doing so, they took care of me too. Then they came back the following March when I was away at a conference, and stayed another week with Eileen.

Even if we hadn't added on to the house, Connie and Karen still would have taken care of Eileen, but now with the addition and the new sofa, they could do it in style! It was something that made Eileen happy, and when you are battling cancer, being happy is the best treatment you can hope for.

Then there was the kitchen.

Eileen loved to cook and entertain, and now she had a double oven and as much granite in the form of countertops as you could get in one room. Then there was the wood flooring and oak cabinets, all designed by Eileen with just a bit of input from me.

By the time Eileen's chemo and radiation treatments were finished, she was ready to hit the kitchen, and it became her focus as she fed her family and friends with her love.

Living the good life helps you live the good life.

It wasn't so much the addition or the new sofa that sustained Eileen and me, but rather, the hope that we indeed could continue to live the good life.

Going to Yankee games and New York Jet games, family movie nights watching our favorite John Candy and Audrey

Hepburn movies, and weekly "May I" card games all helped us continue the life we had always known. Cancer was our bump in the road, and we were lucky to regain control of our lives when the road was smooth again.

I often said that I didn't want to waste my remission. I owed it to other less fortunate patients to not take it for granted. I always had in the back of my mind that it might not always be that way, so I better have fun while I can.

Eileen's mantra had been to go for the best outcome.

She has been lucky, and it wasn't always apparent during her ordeal that she would be, but she continues to live the good life.

Now, make no mistake about it, we continue to have out-of-house experiences. These often include trips to Disney.

Back in 1996 my nephew Michael (my brother Mike's son) and his wife Mary had our whole family down to Disney. They had joined the Disney Vacation Club a year or two before, and they were talking to Mike about taking us down for a trip.

It was a Saturday in January, and Mike called to tell me all about it and said that it would be a year from this coming September. I thought that was great and was very excited. He got off the phone but called me back five minutes later to tell me that instead of next September we could go this September. Mike asked me if this was okay, and I responded that this year or next didn't matter since I wouldn't be able to save either way and that a credit card would be used.

What happened next could be in my Unobtrusive Miracles chapter, because his second phone call was indeed a miracle.

Anyway, we went to Disney in 1996 instead of 1997.

We had a great time, so much so that when we got back, the first thing I did was to purchase a membership in the Disney Vacation Club, and we have been going to Disney every year since.

That second call from Mike telling me we were going in 1996 instead of 1997 was a miracle because we had Mike's funeral that same week in 1997.

Going to Disney took on special meaning to me, and it remains a special place that Eileen and I enjoy. Even though our children don't come down to Disney as often as they used to, they still look forward to leaving the cold of New York for a little Disney magic.

In 2006, Sean, Bryan, my nephew Michael and I went down to Disney and never once went to a theme park. It was spring training that drew us to the friendly confines of Florida. We went to a Yankee spring training game in Tampa and a New York Mets spring training game at Disney's Wild World of Sports.

We were at Disney for three nights, and during that time, we each consumed seven hamburgers. That's what happens when you don't have a woman traveling with you.

To negate this possibility from repeating itself, our trip the next year included Eileen, Karen, and Connie. You might think that traveling with three women would be problematic to a man who had seven hamburgers in three days. You'd be very wrong.

Karen and Connie waited on me hand and foot. My money was no good as they paid for every meal at every restaurant. All they got in return was a place to stay and a pool to sit by and take the occasional plunge.

That first trip was taken in 2008, and we continue to make an annual pilgrimage to Disney, and each year's trip is better than the last.

I had a friend I knew from commuting on the Long Island Rail Road, and he could never understand how I could go to the same place every year. He remarked, "Don't you ever get sick of Mickey Mouse?"

I would have explained to him that it had nothing to do with Mickey, but I knew he wouldn't get it because I had spent the last few years listening to him complain about his trials and tribulations regarding his family, things that were minor in the big picture of life.

Mickey and "all things Disney" were never the attraction for us. It was merely a place where we went with each other as a family and always had a good time. We now expanded the idea of family to include two dear friends. How could you not have a good time when you are sharing the moment with people you love and who love you?

Enjoy The Ride

When we lived in New York, I had an appointment with my hematologist/oncologist three or four times a year, usually on the day when I had one of my monthly IVIG treatments. One time I was told that he wanted to see me between treatments. This raised a red flag in my brain.

I was worried that maybe there was something wrong. Then I told myself that he would have seen me right away if that were the case. Nevertheless, as I drove to Dr. Avvento's Southampton office, I had my worry hat on.

Going to the doctor never really bothers me or causes me any stress, but sometimes I think about the time I took my car in for an oil change and was told my gillhooly rod was out of whack.

My car doesn't have a gillhooly rod and probably yours doesn't either, but mechanics have a language all their own, and I throw myself on their mercy whenever my car is in the shop. So, despite feeling well and anticipating that I would have a good check-up result, I still had a little angst as I drove to my appointment.

I began to wonder what would happen if I were given bad news. How would my view of the world change?

Bucket lists are big these days, and I hate the concept. I have been fortunate in getting just about everything I ever wanted. Of course, a New York Rangers win last night would have really made me happy, but aside from that, I have just about what I need. I don't want to appear to be greedy.

But the thing that scares me most about bucket lists is that they seem so finite. It's a list, after all, and it has a beginning and an end. What happens if you achieve all your list items? Do you merely check out and say so long, everyone?

It's not for me.

I have always subscribed to the concept that wanting is better than having. How many times in our lives have we pursued a goal or a purchase only to achieve our heart's desire and say, "Is that all there is?"

Having an unrealized goal keeps us hungry, keeps us in motion, and keeps us alive.

I won't have a bucket list, but I will see things differently if I get bad news.

It's a short drive from East Quogue to Southampton, but I wasn't even out of Hampton Bays when, talking to myself (it's how I write), I said, "Why do I have to wait for bad news in order to see things differently? Why not let good news help me to see things differently?"

I finished this thought as I approached the village of Southampton. As I passed the Southampton Movie Theater, I noted that *The Fault in Our Stars* was playing.

Oh, bugger!

That only sidetracked me for a second, and I continued my self-examination regarding seeing things differently. I decided that I must change my view of life.

Lately I had bemoaned my commute much more than I ever had done in thirty years. I always was able to put a positive spin on commuting three hours each way every day on the (Very) Long Island Rail Road.

The train was my "den on wheels" where I could read and listen to music and commune with my thoughts. It's where I could write and record my life experiences. I could even have a beer on the ride home. But lately, riding the train had been unbearable.

To honor my newly self-examined self, I vowed that I would enjoy the ride.

Then, as I got deeper into the village, I was just about to "let little things bother me," as my mother always said not to do. It was like a smack at the back of my head when I knew for certain that the train ride was not the only ride I must enjoy.

I longed for the day when my literal train ride would come to an end, and commuting would be a far distant memory. Retirement seemed like a vacation to me. *Maybe it shouldn't*, I mused. *Maybe I shouldn't be so eager to get off the train. Maybe it's the ride that matters most when all is said and done.*

I had a good report from my doctor. In fact, we talked more about the Rangers than we did about me. He said I was doing great, but Nash and Richards needed to score more.

The ride continues, and I mean to enjoy it.

And Yet Here We Are

Did you ever have one of those moments when you realize that your life hasn't turned out quite the way you once thought it would? I have had several.

The most recent was this morning as I rode on the Long Island Rail Road 6:21 out of Speonk. Lately, the last two or three years before I retired, my three-hour door-to-door commute had been getting to me. I used to have a good attitude about commuting six hours a day, but as I'd gotten older, the "good" had diminished, and the "attitude" had lingered.

That morning's attitude was brought on by hearing Harry Chapin's "Cat's in the Cradle." Harry always told a good story in his music, and this song is one of his more poignant renditions. It tells the story of a father and son who are too busy to spend much time with one each other. First, the father is too busy with his job and catching planes and paying bills. Then, the son gets older, and all he wants are the car keys, and eventually his new job is a hassle and the kids have the flu, but he did enjoy talking to his old man on the phone.

Thank God it was Friday.

I have often told my kids not to do what I have done, and the father in the song should feel the same way, but he proudly proclaims, "My boy was just like me."

This song was evocative of another recent experience I had when I saw *Saving Mr. Banks*. During the film, Walt Disney tells a story about holding on to the Mickey Mouse concept when he was just starting out, and this big money guy was looking for something just like Mickey. Disney held on to his idea, and the rest is billion-dollar history. Walt didn't sell out, but I did.

Early in our marriage, my life was much different than the life I now had in East Quogue in the Hamptons. I worked within minutes of my home. I was able to take my newborn son for a walk in the afternoon and play with him in the evening in our New Rochelle basement apartment. But I was making $12,000 a year. This may not seem like much, but the year before I was only making $8,400, and this was a teacher's salary in the late Seventies.

I didn't want to earn $12,000 a year. I didn't want to live in a basement apartment. I wanted to make serious money and live in the Hamptons. I changed jobs and made better if not serious money. We were able to get the house in the Hamptons, and I had a teaching job all set up. Well, the superintendent screwed me over on that one and told me they were going to hire a kid right out of college because they would have to pay me too much. So, here I was with a house in the Hamptons and the lonesome wail of the locomotive waiting at the station. But, eventually, I would get a job out on the east end of Long Island, if only for a few moments.

In the meantime, we had another child, Jeannine, and eventually a third, Bryan. Over the years, I continued to commute, and even went to law school and I eased my commute by living with my father in the Bronx. It's funny, but as I think back, I never remember listening to "Cat's in the Cradle" back then. Maybe if I had, I would have realized what my son Sean realized for me.

I was always beating myself up for "not being there" for my family. The truth is I was there.

I was there for my father. I have no doubt that going back to live with him during the week when I was in law school added years to his life. He had a purpose once more. He had me to take care of, and it was like going back to Leland Avenue for both of us. Then when I went home on Thursday nights, I was there for my wife and kids. The kids were asleep on Thursdays, but when I came home from work on Fridays, I was always packing M&Ms or a Milky Way for each. I was like Bob Cratchit in *A Christmas Carol* coming home with chestnuts.

I realized that "being there" is not a time sensitive activity. You don't have to be in the same room 24/7. But when you are in the same room, you better be there and not somewhere else. When I was at a Yankee game with Sean one time, bemoaning my life and my commute, and the dread I felt at not "being there" for my kids, Sean let me go on and on, and then he replied, "And yet here we are."

So, "Cat's in the Cradle" turns out to be a happy tale after all, but I still wouldn't recommend commuting six hours a day.

Unobtrusive Miracles

One of the many advantages of going to Catholic schools is that you are quite familiar with the concept of miracles.

The trouble is that most of the stories of miracles we're familiar with are in what I like to call the Cecil B. DeMille category — you know, big blockbuster movie miracles with lightning bolts, parted seas, and a booming heavenly voice that sounds uncannily like Charlton Heston's.

The trouble is that we rarely think of the kind of miracles that happen when we are on our way to Damascus and we're struck blind while God talks to us about our errant ways of living. No, sometimes God's voice isn't even much of a whisper.

My first realization of this was back in 1997 when I was trying to come to grips with the loss of my brother Michael. I had prayed every day for nearly three weeks for the type of miracle that would raise him from his sick bed, only to be denied. It was when I was writing his eulogy that I was persuaded to think otherwise.

On that dark day in August of 1997, I was brought back to another day in June of 1966.

Michael was twenty-two and therefore ripe for the Vietnam War that was blazing out of control. He received his draft notice along with the infamous subway token, so he couldn't cop the "I ain't got no money to be traveling down to Whitehall Street" plea.

Of course, he was accepted as a recruit, and would soon be destined for points very Far East if it were not for the first unobtrusive miracle of my experience.

Prior to his Selective Service invite, Michael had applied for service in the Army National Guard. His application was accepted in time, and on the day he would have reported to Whitehall Street, he was sent off to some god-awful place in Maryland for basic training in the Guard.

I realized thirty years later as I wrote his eulogy that Michael had been spared. I realized, too, that the miracle I, and the rest of his family, had been praying for all of August 1997 had actually been granted in June of 1966.

I recently became aware of another unobtrusive miracle.

I had been sick, off and on, pretty much all summer with the cold that never seemed to go away. My CLL had been in remission for about eight years, but lately my white blood cell count had been going up. Still, I was not ready for the next round of treatment. My cold came back, and my numbers kept going up, so my oncologist ordered a PET scan.

Enlarged lymph nodes, enlarged spleen, and all of a sudden I was in for another tonsil biopsy.

I had a similar biopsy in 2007, the last time my CLL was treated. Eileen accompanied me to the procedure and was in the office with me when it was performed, thank God. I don't know what it was. Nerves? The gag reflex gone awry? All I remember is that Eileen and the doctor seemed to change places, and before I knew it, I heard the doctor say, "There he goes."

I only was out for a second — well, Eileen said it was much longer. Anyway, I survived that biopsy, but I have to tell you, thinking of that episode had me just a little bit anxious as I made my way to the doctor's office.

The procedure went well, and I would get the results the following week. But when I got home, an unobtrusive miracle soon made its appearance, and it had absolutely nothing to do with me.

Eileen and I had just finished our lunch when the phone rang. It was my ENT physician, but he was calling Eileen.

I was still a little out of it from the pain medication given me for the biopsy, so I wasn't really paying attention. The fact that Eileen had gotten the call wasn't a surprise. She had been in to see the same doctor for a hearing test earlier in the week, and I just assumed this was a follow-up.

When she got off the phone, she seemed a little relieved — well, if I were paying attention, I would have sensed that. She had to fight for my attention by stating, "The MRI came back negative."

I am dense. And when I have been numbed up, my density only increases. But I finally got it.

"What MRI?"

Eileen then informed me that she'd had an MRI that morning.

My mouth literally fell open. "What? Why?"

"Because there was a concern for a brain tumor."

I was flabbergasted! "How could you keep this from me?"

"You were having the same biopsy that made you pass out on a good day. I wasn't going to take any chances, especially when I didn't know for sure."

She was right of course. After forty years of marriage, she knew exactly what she was doing.

I have to say, though, that it was a moment we often hear described as a near-death experience. Your life appears like a movie on fast forward, and you see all that has happened in your short stay on this planet.

Except, for me, in this moment, it was the future that appeared, or what would have been the future.

We were planning our move to Florida and beginning a new chapter of our life in a new house on the Gulf Coast, free from winter's frigid cold and as close to a tiki bar as I could manage.

But instead of relaxing with Eileen in a nice house with a pool in the lanai, I saw myself alone in a very dark place.

That MRI was the latest in my experience of unobtrusive miracles that washed over me, convincing me that the pool in the lanai might yet be in our future, and in fact, that it *would* be our future. I wouldn't be alone. I wouldn't be in a dark place.

The future is still out there. What kind of future it will be, no one gets a guarantee.

I just thank God for the unobtrusive miracles and hope He continues sending them our way.

Faith, Toys, And Automobiles

I used to be a fan of the TV show *Touched by an Angel.* I guess it was a time in my life when I really needed a little divine intervention. But, as I recall, as soon as I finished watching an episode, I switched to the next entry of *The Sopranos.* Nevertheless, the concept of angels intrigues me still.

Eileen and I had a recent discussion about angels. She is a believer in their existence and involvement in our lives. I believe in them too, and there have been occasions in my life that can only be chalked up to the intervention of angels.

On the first occasion of angel spotting that occurred in my life, I was actually the angel. It was a Sunday evening, and I was driving back to the Bronx after dropping Eileen off at St. Vincent's School of Nursing. I was driving my 1973 Chevy Vega. Having skimped on my car purchase by not buying the Nova, it should be no surprise that I avoided the toll on the Triborough Bridge and went by way of the no toll Madison Avenue Bridge and 138th street. Those of you who have made this maneuver will recall the ramp coming onto 138th and the lovely environs in which you were deposited.

Just as I was coming off the ramp and making the right turn toward the Bruckner Expressway, I saw a stalled car on the side of the road. It was my friend Paul of Pat and Paul fame. He looked at me as I pulled up as if I were a messenger from God. I think I was. I was there just at the right moment. Fifteen minutes earlier and I would have missed him. Had I opted to pay the 50-cent toll, I would have missed him. It was God who determined that I would be late and cheap at the same time. As my wife Eileen is often heard to say, "There are no coincidences."

Fast-forward a couple of years, and in that same 1973 Chevy Vega, Eileen and I were heading into the Bronx from our apartment in Flushing. We were on the Van Wyck heading to the Whitestone Bridge. Just as we approached the bridge, my Vega started acting, well, like a Vega. I was able to goose it up the bridge to the last exit in Queens. As we rolled down the Third Avenue exit in Whitestone, I looked in the rear view mirror and saw Pat and Paul in their car. They just happened to be on their way from Brooklyn to the Bronx, too. They returned the favor that I had extended a few years earlier. There are no coincidences.

The next visitation occurred sometime in the summer of 1977. Still driving that same 1973 Chevy Vega, which I had just picked up from our Irish mechanic, Sean, I stopped off to see my parents at 1261 Leland. Sean was a great mechanic. I asked him how much it would cost to fix my electric rear window defroster, and he replied, "How much could it cost?" I never got a real answer, and I never fixed the defroster.

Anyway, when I was at 1261 Leland, I called my friend PJ to confirm that he was coming out to Flushing so that we could go for a run and thereby justify the beer that we would enjoy afterward, but PJ cancelled. He wasn't up to driving, running, or drinking. I was disappointed, but what the heck?

I set off for Flushing, and as I paid the toll on the Bronx side and revved up my four-cylinder aluminum-block animal of a car, the very thing that had caused me to take the car to Sean in the first place happened again. As I accelerated, the manifold pipe fell out, and the car sounded like one of those juiced-up cars that pop wheelies nine feet in the air. Noise wasn't my only problem as I was now dragging this pipe underneath my chassis. Once again, I got off the Whitestone Bridge at the first exit.

I didn't know what to do so I called PJ. He was tying up my manifold pipe fifteen minutes later despite the fact that he had been too tired to drive, run, or drink. Now most people would just see this as an extremely nice thing done by an extremely good friend. I used to think that, and in fact, I used this example of friendship in the religion class I taught at St. Vito's. Had I known better, I would have said that PJ was an angel that night, but he never knew it, and until recently, neither did I.

For the next angelic tale, we really have to go back to the future. I was working at Columbia and still looking to go back into teaching. I had an interview somewhere in the town of Islip. I drove to work in those days, and my car was a 1975 Mercury Monarch. We bought this eight-cylinder beast that was bad on gas twelve hours before the gasoline crisis of 1979 started.

Anyway, it was now 1985, and the car was on its last legs.

It didn't have a check engine light as such but one that when lit stated, "You're killing me, you bastard."

So, here I was driving onto the Southern State Parkway near Babylon, and my Monarch abdicates and goes and dies on me. I get to the shoulder and immediately a trooper comes and calls in for a tow truck. Not two minutes later, I see a car pull off to the side of the highway, and out of it comes my nephew Jimmy.

"Uncle Jimmy, what's going on?"

Well, Jimmy was driving his parents' car, as they were away on a European vacation. Jimmy drove me to the repair shop where we held a funeral service for the Monarch, and then we went to his home in Baldwin. He gave me the keys to the car and told me it was mine to drive for the week.

How did my nephew arrive just at the moment when I needed to be rescued? There are no coincidences.

There have been other instances of divine intervention that may be considered mere coincidence, but I know better. Two people starting to say the same thing at the same time is a coincidence.

People who just happen to appear out of nowhere when you need them most?

You decide.

It was Christmas Eve 1985. Sean was four and Jeannine would soon turn two. The setting is the pediatric ward of Southampton Hospital. Sean's asthma was acting up, and he could not tolerate the medicine when taken orally so he had to be admitted so that an IV drip could be administered. Our good friends Marybeth and Leo watched Jeannine for us as Eileen and I settled in for a Christmas Eve in the hospital.

Sean was the only kid in pediatrics, and Santa was making a special trip to visit him. As he approached the room, Eileen and I bolted out to head him off before Sean saw him. I guess we startled poor Santa when we said as forcefully as we could without shouting, "It is NOT Christmas Eve!"

Well, poor Santa didn't understand at first, but then we explained that we intended to have Christmas on the 26th and

Christmas Eve, therefore, on the 25th when Sean would be going home.

The hospital staff played along with us and made sure no one said that Santa was coming tonight, and we changed TV channels anytime we sensed anything that might expose our lie. However, Sean did see one commercial for a toy that would have a tremendous impact on our night and our lives.

There was a cartoon show that Sean liked in those days, *ThunderCats*, and their vehicle was the ThunderTank. Well, as he was watching the commercial for the ThunderTank, he turned to Eileen and me and said, "I sure hope Santa gives me that for Christmas." I looked at Eileen, and she gave me a furtive shake of the head indicating that Santa had come up empty as far as the ThunderTank was concerned.

I was going out to get Sean McDonald's for dinner, and Eileen suggested that I try the two toy stores in Southampton. There was no way these small shops would have something that Toys R Us or Child World didn't have, but I said I would try.

I could see that Toy World was already closed, so I drove to McDonald's and got Sean his Happy Meal. It was around 4:45 when I left McDonald's and I drove a few blocks out of my way just in case Lillywhite's Toy Store was still open. It was.

Lillywhites was a quaint, old-fashioned toy store. There were no video games to be had here, but you could probably still get a Tinkertoy. It was nearly 5:00 p.m., and closing time was fast approaching. Rather than search the shelves, I headed straight for the counter where a young woman was standing. I asked her if she had heard of a ThunderTank, and she replied, "Sure, there is one right behind you."

I felt like George Bailey! Here it was Christmas Eve, and I was able to get the one toy that my son, who was sick in the hospital on Christmas Eve, so wanted Santa to bring. It was amazing.

Not wishing to let this poor girl go home without me telling her about my son in the hospital, I gushed the whole thing out as I deposited my Mastercard on the counter. She looked up at me and rather sheepishly said, "I'm sorry, sir, but we don't take credit cards."

Despair, frustration, anger all competed for my attention. I just could not believe it. I had cash back at the hospital, but I didn't have time to go get it before the store closed. Of course, in the real world, Christmas was tomorrow and I would be unable to get it then. I was lost and beaten.

Now children, if you ever doubted that there really was a Santa Claus, I am about to tell you why you are seriously wrong.

In the pit of despair, when I was just about coming to grips that my mission had failed, I saw in the corner of my eye some type of motion in the back room of the store. I looked up and an elderly woman was gingerly approaching the store counter. She looked at me and the young lady who was trying to help me, and asked what the trouble was.

The girl explained, "This man wants to buy this toy for his son, but he only has a credit card."

The old woman said, "So what is the problem? We'll bill him." I couldn't believe my ears.

"I'm sorry, what did you say?" I asked, needing clarification.

She replied, "We will send you a bill, and you will pay for the toy when you get the bill." Even as I type this, I get goose bumps. Where in the world in 1986 would this ever happen? No mega store, no chain, no big box store would ever let you leave the premises with anything that wasn't paid for in full, and here this kind woman from another generation came to my rescue.

For several Christmas Eves after this one, I visited Lillywhites to buy at least one toy. While shopping in the store, I would re-tell this story to some poor soul who happened to make eye contact with me that day.

So, I went back to the hospital, Sean had his Happy Meal, and I had to go home to put the ThunderTank together. Sean came home the next day, and Santa came that night, but you couldn't convince me that Santa hadn't come the day before in a small store in Southampton. Yes, I really do believe in Santa Claus, and you should too.

There have been many angels in our lives and none so loving as when we were dealing with cancer. Family, friends, and colleagues all had our back and kept us strong.

We're All On This Journey Together

In January 2017, Eileen and I moved down to Bradenton, Florida. Of course, we left a great deal behind. Sean, Jeannine, and Bryan are still in New York, and there isn't a day that we don't wish they were down here with us.

I have retired, and many people have asked how I am adjusting. Well, not having the kids around has been the hardest thing to adjust to.

Just the day before I wrote this, Eileen and I met with our local oncologist. Once again, we have struck gold. He and his staff are terrific, and were so attentive to both of us and listened to our history like it really mattered to them.

Health-wise, Eileen and I are doing well. I have resumed taking Ibrutinib, and my white blood cell counts have continued to show positive results. Eileen is feeling well and is on a schedule to see our new oncologist every six months.

The journey that Eileen and I began in August of 2000 when I was first diagnosed seems to have been a very long one. This entire millennium, our lives have been impacted by cancer. I am not sure that back then I would have believed that I would still be here today in 2018. Being told when you are fifty that you have a good ten-year prognosis isn't very encouraging, but here I am.

Then, in 2010, when Eileen's journey with breast cancer began, I had no reason to believe that she would be here eight years later. I never let myself think otherwise, but still, you hear so many sad stories when you are a member of the cancer community.

There remain times when, against the advice of my mother, I do let little things bother me. In those moments, Eileen reins me in and reminds me how lucky I am.

It can be annoying, especially because she is always right.

So many of us are struggling with this disease, and none of us should be alone. None should have to bear this burden alone.

Be sure to talk to people even if it is not directly related to your cancer. As Eileen has pointed out, the human touch can be the most powerful medicine.

Thank you for joining us on our journey. If you enjoyed this book and felt that it touched your life in some way, we would appreciate a great review on Amazon.

More than anything, we would love to hear from you. We invite you to visit our website at www.marriedwithcancer.net.